HIGH-FUNCTIONING AUTISM
A FOUR DECADE JOURNEY AND MEMOIR

HIGH-FUNCTIONING AUTISM
A FOUR DECADE JOURNEY AND MEMOIR

ROBERT MARSHALL BOYER
Self-Advocate with High-Functioning Autism

with TERESA BRYANT GENTRY

KRB PUBLISHING
A KRB ART & RESIN CRAFTS
COMPANY

© 2021 Robert Marshall Boyer

All rights reserved. No part of this publication may be reproduced, distributed, or transmitted in any form or by any means -- photocopying, recording, scanning, electronic, mechanical or other -- except in the case of brief quotations embodied in critical reviews or articles without the prior written permission of the publisher.

Author has tried in good faith to recreate events, locales, and conversations from his memories of them. To protect privacy, in some instances Author may have, but not limited to changing the names of individuals and places, changing some identifying characteristics and details such as physical properties, occupations and places of residence.

Author has made in good faith every effort to ensure that the information in this book was correct at press time, the author does not assume and hereby disclaims any liability to any party for any loss, damage, or disruption caused by errors or omissions, whether such errors or omissions result from negligence, accident, or any other cause.

This book is not intended as a substitute for the medical advice of physicians. The reader should consult a physician in matters relating to his/her health and particularly with respect to any symptoms that may require diagnosis or medical attention.

Any registered trademarks, including on photographs, mentioned in the memoir are owned by the respected owners, and Author does not claim ownership or rights to the trademarks that are mentioned inside the memoir. Any photographs provided inside the memoir comes from the personal private collection of the Author, claiming personal rights to the photographs, which may include professional photos such as Olan Mills ® that provided services for professional grade photos.

Any Internet Addresses, phone numbers, or company or product information printed in this book are offered as a resource and are not intended in any way to be or to imply an endorsement by KRB Publishing, nor does KRB Publishing vouch for the existence, content, or services of these sites, phone numbers, companies, or products beyond the life of this book.

The Front Book Cover designed by Robert Marshall Boyer with an Olan Mills ® photograph of Robert Marshall Boyer.

Additional Author, Teresa Bryant Gentry
Consulting Editor, Karen Ray Boyer, RN

ISBN: 978-0-578-86008-4

Library of Congress Cataloging-in-Publication Data
Library of Congress Control Number: 2021903464

Printed in the United States of America

KRB Publishing, P.O. BOX 21, McLeansville, NC 27301-0021

A SPECIAL ACKNOWLEDGEMENT TO TERESA BRYANT GENTRY

This personal memoir is dedicated to my mother, Teresa. She was the one who kept many health-related records such as auditory hearing studies, psychological evaluations, medical evaluations, Individualized Education Plan (IEP) records and North Carolina Vocational Rehabilitation (VR) records from the span that started from 1987 to the early 2000s. With her dedication and knowledge, she felt the need to keep these important documents. Her hard work taught me by word and deed to collect all my health-related records from the early 2000s throughout the process of my autism diagnosis from mid-2019 to February 2020.

IN MEMORIAM OF J. MARSHALL BRYANT

My Grandfather, Joseph Marshall Bryant, helped shape me into who I am. He helped me understand my abilities, which helped enhance and strengthen me into the person I am. From the beginning, my grandfather, simply known as "Marshall," to all those who loved him, helped to channel my narrow, obsessive-like interests with wildlife, NASCAR, other sports, his military services, and other interests over the years. He did not know at the time how he shaped my interests for the better; I like to say they are passions *not* obsessions. He knew I was socially awkward all of my life, so he was trying to help me, be patient with me, and build and work on my social issues. I'm not sure that he completely knew what was going on, other than I had a diagnosis of auditory processing, learning disabilities and AD/HD deficits, and other issues from early evaluations. I considered him my best friend in many aspects throughout my life, as long as we were blessed to have him.

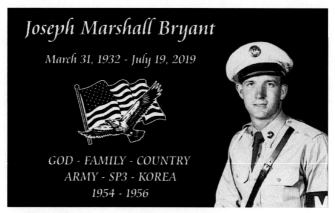

Foot Stone Marker (digital) of Joseph Marshall Bryant. Gifted from Robert Marshall Boyer to Mr. Bryant's children and family.

For all of those who are struggling with autism-like developmental issues that have been misdiagnosed, underdiagnosed, or have not been diagnosed, this is for you!

There is hope, no matter how long your journey will take. I still struggle daily, but to help those who continue to struggle, I wanted to share my journey with you. -Robert M. Boyer.

TABLE OF CONTENTS

Introduction	1
The Two Subtypes of Autism	5
1 Birth to Fifth Grade	11
2 Middle and High School	37
3 Summer 1999 to Summer 2000	49
4 July 2002 to June 23, 2012	67
5 July 2012 to May 29, 2019	85
6 Fully Disabled with Autism	103
Autism Diagnosis & DNA Testing	107
Facts About Autism From the National Autism Association	111
Questions and Answers Section: With Robert Marshall Boyer	113
About the Authors/Editor	121

HIGH-FUNCTIONING AUTISM

INTRODUCTION

There were two subtypes of autism until 2012, but things changed in 2013. The original subtypes of autism were established in the mid-20th Century in Europe and the United States from two German-speaking Austrian doctors called psychiatrist pediatricians from 1943 to 1944. At the same time, there was a raging war that was happening across the global stage that hindered things with autism, in part, of language and translation barriers. Many professionals and pioneers researched and reviewed the case studies of these two Austrian child psychiatrists over the following years, but more so in the last four to five decades in the field of autism when some of the studies were translated from German to English. However, from the mid-1970s to 2012, the two subtypes of autism were still separated due to certain types of behavior and symptoms. But things changed in 2013 inside the field of autism.

One subtype of autism was less severe than the other autism subgroup, but both had many of the same mechanisms. The mild version of autism included a more intelligent background, but still lacked social skills and communication skills. The severe version of autism needed supporting help from the health system, community, and family. The severe version of autism was known as, "classic autism."

HIGH-FUNCTIONING AUTISM

Over the years, the subtypes of autism were called by different names. From the mid-1970s to 2012, their formal names were called Asperger's syndrome, but also known as Asperger's Disorder (Asperger's) in recent diagnosis manuals and classic autism (Autism). However, both subtypes would merge into one umbrella of diagnosis under the formal diagnosis term called Autism Spectrum Disorder (ASD), beginning in the year 2013, which all autistic-related diagnosis were labeled into different forms and support levels of ASD. This memoir will focus on real life events based on memories from family, friends, educators, healthcare providers in association of healthcare and educational documents collected, and saved over the years by Teresa Bryant Gentry, and what makes up the developmental and health file of Robert Marshall Boyer, which would have helped him being diagnosed with Asperger's prior to the year 2013.

Since the year 2013, Asperger's is now defined as the mildest form of autism called high-functioning autism (HFA) in the umbrella of Autism Spectrum Disorder. It is in the Level 1 Support category. These individuals are intelligent with a normal to above intelligence quotient (IQ). They do excel in their overall academic studies and employment in some shape or form, but some do still fall through the cracks due to impairments.

Those with HFA struggle with milder impairments of social skills, communication, and language skills. Their deficits start to become more of an issue as they age in their preteen childhood, causing them to not keep up with the expectations of their family and extended community social circles.

HIGH-FUNCTIONING AUTISM

In the case of Robert "Bobby" Boyer and his undiagnosed HFA, he had a complexity of underlying developmental, learning disabilities and mental issues that caused his undiagnosed autism to become worse over his life span, even after he was diagnosed at age 39 years, four months old in February of 2020. We will get into the other issues in this memoir later. Nevertheless, Mr. Boyer continues to struggle like other autism individuals in the spectrum.

In recent decades, many children have become misdiagnosed, underdiagnosed, or never diagnosed with the less severe subtype of autism, creating less quality of life for this group of children, and these individuals would lack needed resources when they went from childhood to adulthood. This important fact does apply to the undiagnosed autism case of Mr. Boyer. He was born during the time that Asperger's studies were getting more well known in many English-speaking countries, but it would take 11 years before Asperger's was thrown in the spotlight and introduced in healthcare diagnosis manuals, and it would take an additional 12 years before Asperger's would become part of the umbrella of Autism Spectrum Disorder. By the time Asperger's became high-functioning autism in 2013, Mr. Boyer was approaching 23-years-old.

On October 16, 1980, Robert Marshall Boyer was born to the parents of Teresa Bryant and Michael Boyer in Burlington, North Carolina.

This memoir will share Mr. Boyer's journey that took a span of nearly four decades to receive a proper diagnosis of Autism Spectrum Disorder.

HIGH-FUNCTIONING AUTISM

HIGH-FUNCTIONING AUTISM

THE TWO SUBTYPES OF AUTISM

The term Asperger's syndrome, the milder version of autism, was a relatively new diagnosis in the field of autism and was named in honor of Hans Asperger (Asperger), a German-speaking Austrian psychiatrist and pediatrician. He was best known for his Writing on *Autistic Psychopathy* that was, and still is, an *Enpony of Asperger's syndrome*.

Asperger, who was born on February 18, 1906 in the German-speaking city of Vienne, Austria, was the director of the University Children's Clinic in Vienna. He spent most of his professional life in his place of birth, publishing autistic case studies in the German language.

Forty-nine years earlier, a Swiss psychiatrist named Paul Eugen Bleuler (Bleuler) was born on April 30, 1857 in Zollikon, Switzerland. He was known for coining the terms *schizophrenia, schizoid and autism.*

In 1910, Bleuler used the term "autismus" that means "autism" in English. He defined autism as a morbid, self-admiration symptom of schizophrenia.

Asperger adopted Bleuler's terminology of "autistic psychopaths" starting in 1938 in child psychology lectures inside Vienna University Hospital. It does appear that the second definition of "autism" came from Asperger between 1938 to 1944, during the raging war of World War II.

During World War II, Asperger was studying only four young boys in his clinic. He saw a pattern of behavior and

HIGH-FUNCTIONING AUTISM

abilities, calling it "autistic psychopathy." The two words translate to "self personality" in non-scientific terms.

Inside the publication in 1944, Asperger noted certain patterns in the four boys that described the boys of having a difficulty in integrating themselves socially, lack of nonverbal communication, but their intelligence appeared to be normal to above normal. However, they had a lack of empathy with their peer group that caused a lack of forming normal friendships. In addition, they had many one-sided conversations that were either disjointed in nature that at times were overly formal with intensive narrow, obsessive-like topics, and interests, and at the same time they were clumsy-natured, which caused them to be socially awkward around their peers, family and the public. However, Asperger called them "little professors" because they had the ability to have an all-absorbing interest in any single topic, and they would dominate their conversations. Nevertheless, he believed these four boys would have the capability of exceptional achievements with original thoughts, sometime later in their life.

Just a year before the 1944 publication of Doctor Asperger's studies of the four boys, there was another child psychiatrist named Leo Kanner (Kanner). He was studying another subtype of autism and published his findings in 1943. Kanner was an Austrian-Hungry native who was born on June 13, 1894. He is best known as the *Father of Child Psychiatry*. When he immigrated to the United States of America in 1924, he described a similar syndrome like Doctor Asperger's cases in a 1943 publication of autistic studies. His autism case study descriptions would be defined as "classic autism" or "Kannerian autism."

Kannerian autism at the time, and still is a classic hallmark that describes the "classic autism" criteria. Any individuals with this severe form of autism will have significant cognitive and communicative deficiencies, including delayed or absent language development deficiencies, which were focused on the developmental approach of Arnold Gesell,

HIGH-FUNCTIONING AUTISM

while Doctor Asperger's autism case studies were influenced by the accounts of schizophrenia and personality disorders, which were in reference of the Eugen Bleuler's typology, in which Asperger's accounts were described as "penetrating but not sufficiently systematic."

The two Austrian-born child psychiatrists studied two ends of the autism spectrum independently in their lifetime. Doctor Hans Asperger was unaware of Doctor Leo Kanner's autism description that was published in 1943, a year before Asperger's autistic description was published in 1944. The world itself was at a different place and time due to the Atlantic Ocean separating Europe and America, including a raging world war, and more importantly, Asperger's autism descriptions were ignored in North America because his studies were all in the German language. His studies would remain largely unknown outside the German-speaking world, but that changed in the late 20th Century.

In the 1970s, Doctor Hans Asperger's autism studies were getting even more attention in English-speaking countries like the United Kingdom (UK) between the mid-1970s to the early 1980s, but Doctor Asperger's description of autism would begin to take notice in the United States of America by the 1990s.

Based on Ishikawa and Ichihashi in the *Japanese Journal of Clinical Medicine*, Gerhard Bosch (Bosch), who was a psychiatrist and a professor at Frankfurt University, used "Asperger's syndrome" for the first time in an English literature on the autism studies that was called *Infantile Autism*. It was first printed in his native tongue of German in 1962. However, it took eight more years to translate and print the book into English. Inside the groundbreaking book about infantile autism, he described his monograph by detailing five case histories that were related to the subgroup of autism called pervasive developmental disorders (PDD). His book would be the first German established research on the field of autism, focusing on toddlers and younger children, and it got attention from professional peers outside the German-speaking world.

In a 1981 series of autism case study publications, an English child psychiatrist named Lorna Gladys Wing (Wing) popularized the term "Asperger's syndrome." She was best known for her important work in *childhood developmental disorders, autism spectrum diagnosis, and Asperger's syndrome.*

Wing was born in Gillingham, Kent, England. In the early 1960s she helped found the National Autistic Society (NAS) in the UK in 1962.

One of her major accomplishments in her career was the first ever role in popularizing the autistic subtype term that would become "Asperger's syndrome" that paid respect from Asperger's work. She helped bring his studies into the English-speaking healthcare community with a 1981 case series about her research in autism studies, which showed similar behaviors and symptoms that were first noted and observed by Doctor Hans Asperger in the mid-1940s.

Therefore, Wing placed Asperger's syndrome into the autism spectrum. However, the difference between Wing's point of view and Asperger's point of view were much different. Doctor Asperger did not feel comfortable in characterizing his patients on the continuum of autism spectrum disorders. Therefore, and out of respect of the early studies of Doctor Asperger, and to avoid any misunderstanding as a neutral term, and using the term "autistic psychopathy" with a sociopathic behavior, she honored Doctor Asperger's pioneering work for this subtype of autism by labeling all her case studies as "Asperger's syndrome."

Doctor Wing's Asperger's syndrome case study research, and other related work, started to influence her professional peers to think some similar thoughts on this subtype of autism. Nevertheless, her interpretation and observation blurred distinctions between studies from Doctor Asperger

HIGH-FUNCTIONING AUTISM

and Doctor Kanner. Unlike her peers before her, she included some children with intellectual disabilities and children with language delays early in their lives, which can be interrupted to the moderate level of the three levels of the current ASD diagnosis. Her work would heavily influence the diagnostic concept of American psychiatry, and "Asperger's syndrome" would simply become Asperger's.

The first systematic studies of Asperger's (high-function autism) appeared in three different publications in Europe and North America in the late 1980s. The first one in the UK by *Tantam* (1988). The second one in Sweden by *Gillberg and Gilbert* (1989). The third one in North American by *Szatmari, Bartolucci and Bremmer* (1989). Out of the three studies from 1988 and 1989, *Gillberg and Gillberg* (1989) shared the diagnostic criteria for Asperger's syndrome, which *Szatmari* (1989) also proposed the same criteria of diagnosis.

In 1991, a book written called *Autism and Asperger's Syndrome*, written by a German developmental psychologist Uta Frith (Frith), was the first book in English about the term Asperger's syndrome. With the background and special interest in autism and dyslexia, Frith believed these conditions were of "psychogenic" origin by linking them to the brain and behavior. That thought of thinking changed the mainstream view in the professional field of autism about the two brain disorders, as her research continued to grow and influence her professional peers. Two main theories in her career explained the core issues of autism that was "lack of implicit mentalizing" and 'weak central coherence." What is Implicit mentalizing? It is the automatic ability to predict behavior from moment to moment on the basis of mental states such as beliefs and desires. What is weak central coherence? It is the ability of focusing on fine detail but failing to see the bigger picture. Therefore, weak central coherence can give rise to some special talents within the high-functioning autism individuals. Due to Frith's contribution, Asperger's became a formal diagnostic in healthcare manuals, starting in the mid-

HIGH-FUNCTIONING AUTISM

1990s.

Starting in 1992, Asperger's syndrome became a distinct diagnosis when it was included in the 10th published edition of the *World Health Organization's diagnostic manual* and the *International Classification of Diseases (ICD-10)*. Two years later, in 1994, it was added to the fourth edition of the *Diagnostic and Statistical Manual of Mental Disorders (DSM-IV)* as Asperger's Disorder.

Since the widespread introduction of Asperger's into the English-speaking audience, there are many sources on the topic, ranging from hundreds of books, articles and websites that describe it, dramatically increasing the awareness for Autism Spectrum Disorder, which at one point it was recognized as an important subgroup with a current debate of concerns. Inside the peer groups of the field of autism, there was a debate on whether it should be a separate condition from high-functioning autism, but this fundamental issue required further study. There was some tentative and little consensus among clinical researchers about the usage of the term "Asperger's syndrome" about the empirical validation of the *DSM-IV* and *ICD-10* criteria. It has been debated that the definition of the condition will change as new studies emerge, eventually being understood as a multifactorial heterogeneous neurodevelopmental disorder that would involve a chemical change, resulting in prenatal or perinatal changes in brain structures. As it would come to pass, the *DSM-V* in 2013 placed Asperger's among other autism-like conditions into one umbrella called Autism Spectrum Disorder, creating a better situation to get federal help in resources in the United States, which prior to 2013, Asperger's did not qualify for federal help for individuals and their caregivers or family.

CHAPTER 1
BIRTH TO FIFTH GRADE

During the pregnancy and labor process in early to middle of 1980, my mother was struggling. She had suffered with nausea and vomiting that haunted her throughout her first trimester and took Bendectin (also Doxylamine/pyridoxine), which later was discontinued in 1982-1983 due to the allegations that it caused congenital malformations. Studies found an increase in chances of limb reduction defects, oral clefts, and diaphragmatic hernias, which is based on the website *Birth Defect Research for Children* on their website section *www.birthdefects.org/bendectin*. In addition, she hemorrhaged, and it was noted from verbal conversations that I had a, "big head," and I was, stuck in the birth canal during my birth, and it was too late to do a Cesarean Section delivery. Therefore, the medical team had to use forceps to pull my head out of the birth canal. My birth weight was about seven and a half pounds. Thankfully, no neonatal issues came up the first weeks after birth. They named me Robert Marshall after my father's middle name, and the first name of my fraternal grandfather and uncle, and my middle name came from my maternal grandfather's middle name.

HIGH-FUNCTIONING AUTISM

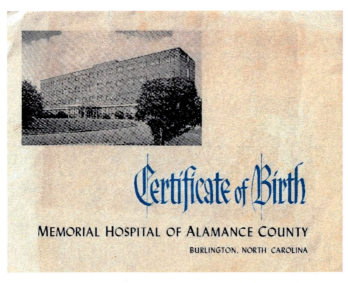

Photocopy of Certificate of Birth of Robert. He was seven pounds, four ounces with a length of 20 inches (document not shown).

HIGH-FUNCTIONING AUTISM

From what I know, my biological father had speech therapy, and was later diagnosed with dyslexia in his 20s. His background includes occasional obsessive-like behaviors, being an artistic person and having normal to above normal intelligence. He was never diagnosed with any form of autism spectrum disorder that I am aware of.

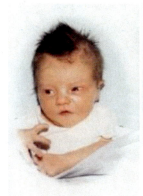

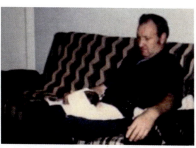

Above: Robert. Less than a week old with Marshall, maternal grandfather.

Top Left: Robert, October 18, 1980. Two-Days Old.

Below: Robert's First Birthday Party, October 1981 with Marshall. At the home of Ruby Bryant, great-aunt.

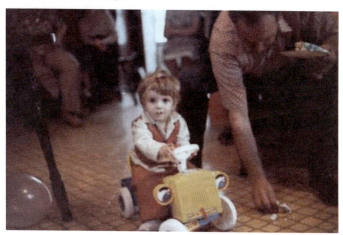

HIGH-FUNCTIONING AUTISM

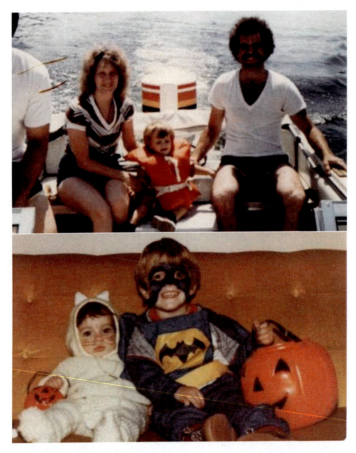

Above: In the summer of 1982. Teresa, Robert and Mike. Olympia, Washington. Visiting Paternal Grandparents and Aunt's Family.

Below: Seresa Marie Boyer, age six months, the sister of Robert, age three. Sometime in October during the Halloween Season of 1983. Robert was, and still is, a big fan of Batman.

    My mother never had any healthcare documentation of mental health diagnoses on herself, prior to my 1987 documentation, which is based on my audiological evaluation

HIGH-FUNCTIONING AUTISM

notes from the audiologist.

By six months of age, I was a happy baby. I sat up and walked before twelve months. I spoke my first words before I turned one-year-old. By age two, I could form two-to-three-word sentences. Between age two and three I was potty trained.

Late 1980 or early 1981. Robert, less than six months old, with Teresa and Mike.

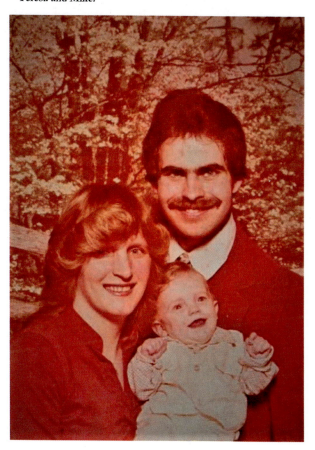

HIGH-FUNCTIONING AUTISM

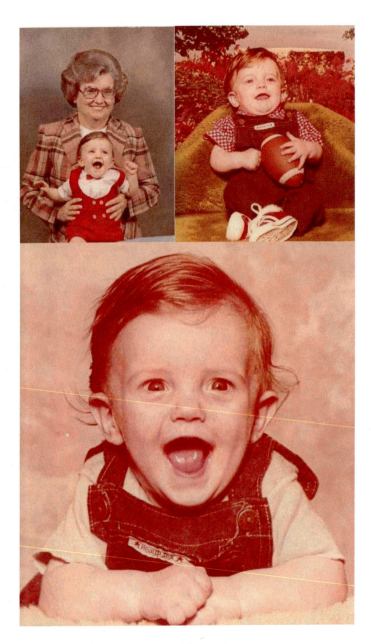

HIGH-FUNCTIONING AUTISM

Previous page of photos includes Top Left: March 1981. Robert, age five months old, with great-aunt, Ruby (sister of Marshall). Top Right and Bottom: April 1981. Robert, age six and a half months old.

Below: October 1982, First Birthday photograph, Robert.

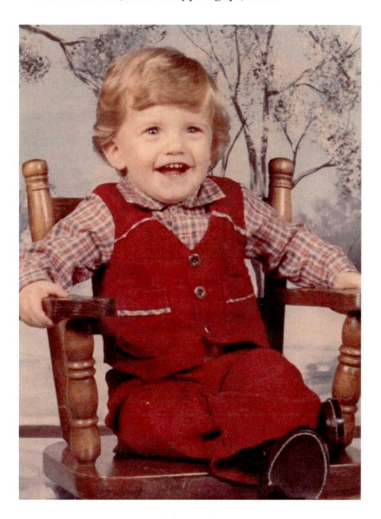

HIGH-FUNCTIONING AUTISM

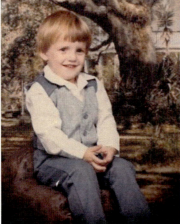

In 1982. Robert, age two years old. The cowboy outfit, one of many outfits provided by his great-aunt Ruby.

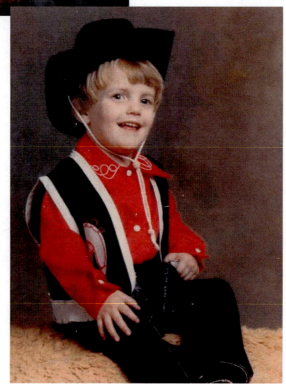

HIGH-FUNCTIONING AUTISM

On April 30, 1983, my little sister was born in Burlington, North Carolina. I loved my baby sister, Seresa Marie. Her first name came from our mother, but replaced the "T" with a "S" in her first name, and her middle name came from her two grandmothers and paternal aunt. Our age gap is only two years and six and a half months in age. Due to our proximity in age, our relationship grew close over the years.

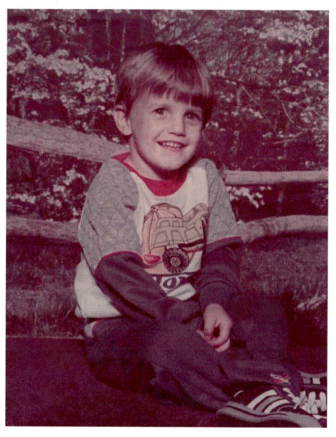

In 1983. Robert, age three years old. Beginning to have development issues with language and speech.

HIGH-FUNCTIONING AUTISM

In healthcare documents, a few years after my birth, it is stated that I did not have any seizures or any major illnesses. However, I was clumsy for the first three years of my life, resulting in minor scrapes and cuts due to many falls. At times I would suffer blows to the head, and at three years of age, I had to get stitches in my forehead. From verbal conversations and a blurred, traumatic memory of that time, I knew that I had hit my forehead and memories of being strapped down in the hospital bed during the process of getting stitched up by the doctor. It was told to me by my mother that I had been, "running in the house when it was dark from what may have been a power outage," or for some reason it was, "dark in the house." Due to my clumsiness and unaware nature, I ran into the side of the doorway opening and busted open my forehead, requiring stitches.

Despite my clumsy nature, I could still ride a bicycle. However, some of my overall motor skills, like tying my shoelaces, was delayed until around six-years of age.

It was reported that I was suspected to have allergies but no signs of Otitis Media (middle ear infection or inflammation). However, it was noted that I had "frequent bouts of coughing and upper respiratory infections, and my parents wondered if I had respiratory allergies."

During my pre-school years to the end of first grade (1982-88), I had sleep disturbance issues. I had many episodes of sleep walking, but no evidence of parasomnias (abnormal movements, behaviors, emotions, perceptions, or dreams). In addition, I had difficulty falling asleep and staying asleep. From 1987 to 1988, I did not have trouble going to sleep, but if I were given permission to fall asleep, I would go to sleep in a classroom setting, frequently. When not allowed to fall asleep, I seemed like I was burnt out easily as "if [I] had been 'running wide open' continuously" with a complaint of being tired in the classroom or in a home environment.

HIGH-FUNCTIONING AUTISM

One of a many red flags of possible autism-like issues over the years, prior to 1988, which was stated in the 1988 evaluation report that noted, "Bobby's behavior despite improvement continues to include much whining, over-reaction to stimuli, and defiance. Bobby is the type of child who always needed someone to play with and keep him entertained. He appeared restless and easily bored. However, he has difficulty participating in large groups."

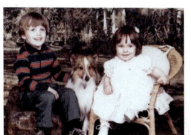

Left: In 1984. Robert and Seresa with their four-year-old dog, Lady, a Scotland Shetland Sheepdog breed also known as "Shelties."

Bottom: Robert, Fourth Birthday Picture. October 1984.

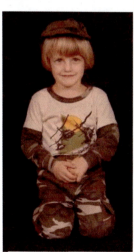
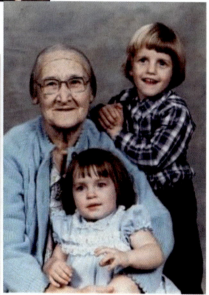

Right Bottom: Christmas 1984. Robert with maternal Great Grandmother Susie Mabe Bryant, age 79, and Seresa, age 19 months.

HIGH-FUNCTIONING AUTISM

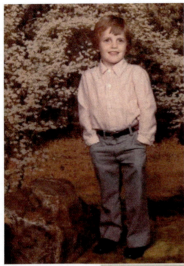

In 1985. Robert, between age four and five years old.

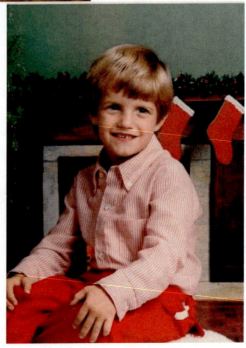

HIGH-FUNCTIONING AUTISM

In addition to this first of many red flags in the 1988 evaluation, this next noted statement backs up the study and theories of Doctor Asperger about narrow, obsessive-like knowledge of single topics of interest, and the working theory of Doctor Frith about weak central coherence, which is the ability of focusing on fine detail but failing to see the bigger picture. Therefore, weak central coherence can give rise to some special talents within the high-functioning autism individuals. The noted documentation in 1988 stated that "Bobby is reported to have difficulty concentrating for even a short period of time unless it is something he really wants to do. When doing a task, he is often careless, unpredictable in his performance, and hurried. He is easily distracted by unimportant details and remembers things that are of little consequences while forgetting the important details."

In the beginning of 1985, I was four and a half years old and took the separation and divorce of my parents extremely hard. I witnessed negative events involving my parents. Also, while my mother was dating other men and the relationships failed, they stated that I tried to comfort my mother to make her feel better during her crying spells from all these post-divorce relationships.

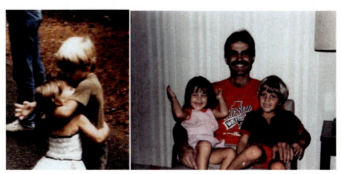

August of 1985, weekend with father. Robert, age four years, 10 months, with his dad Mike and sister, Seresa, age two years, four months.

HIGH-FUNCTIONING AUTISM

Sometime in 1985, during the separation and divorce period, my maternal grandmother Hilda Bryant was picking me up at a daycare for a private speech therapy session. When my grandmother went to the front desk of the daycare, they could not find me inside the building, but it turned out that the daycare had left me, at age four and a half, in their hot daycare van for approximately one hour. They had no clue where I was until they discovered I was missing, and the staff looked in the van where I was sleeping. I'm not sure how I survived that. Someone was looking over me. At the time, my mother was so swamped and overwhelmed being a single mother of two young children, heading to a finalized divorce, that she never had a thought about taking legal action. Thinking back to the seriousness of the event she knows that it possibly contributed to additional neurological damage and development issues later in my life.

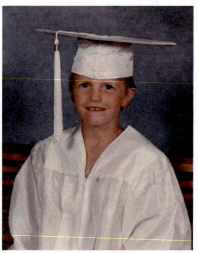

PRE-SCHOOL GRADUATION
JUNE 1986
Robert Boyer
(age five years, eight months old)

HIGH-FUNCTIONING AUTISM

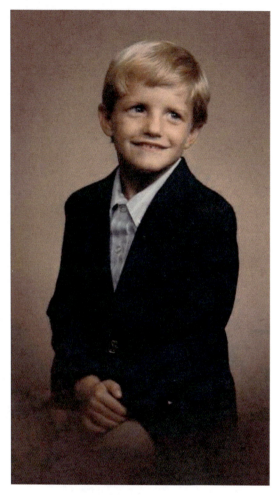

October 1986. Sixth Birthday Party photograph from Olan Mills ® taken of Robert.

From 1985 to 1987, my mental and emotional behavior continued to get worse, in part, related to the separation and divorce of my parents. However, that was about to change when James Watkins Gentry came into my life between 1987 and 1988. Through my mother's first cousin, Phillip

Poteat, she ended up meeting her second husband. Phillip had a house party sometime in 1987. My mother had already known her second husband as a former student at Cummings High School, nearly ten years earlier when he was a drafting teacher, football, and track coach. But she had never had him as a teacher. But, if the verbal conversations and memory are right, she may have been in his homeroom at one point in high school. But, the important thing, she knew whom Mr. Gentry was due to the connections of Teresa being her class's salutatorian and other extracurricular activities in high school.

Due to the inclusion of Mr. Gentry dating my mother, I started to adapt and respond well to a new male figure in my mother's life, causing my negative behavior to reduce in some frequency. My mother believed that my behavior changes were the positive influence of Mr. Gentry, and the added discipline skills she used on me.

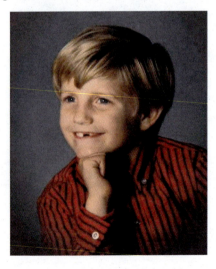

Early October 1987. Seventh Birthday Party Olan Mills ® photograph of Robert.

HIGH-FUNCTIONING AUTISM

On November 13, 1987, at age seven, I was seen by an audiologist for an auditory processing evaluation by the request of a speech pathologist. In an open classroom setting with the audiologist, I was left-handed. It was reported that, I "was not very active," and, "somewhat disorganized," with, "trouble turning the pages of a picture book in a smooth manner.

The findings of the audiological evaluations are as defined below:

    a) Normal bilateral hearing sensitivity, however, mild discrimination difficulties during quiet. Had significant auditory processing difficulties characterized by:
        i) Poor auditory attention with background was present. Exhibited poor skills in discriminating words, focusing attention or maintaining attention on verbal information when auditory distractions were present. This caused difficulties in the classroom when the teacher was talking when other background noise was present. He had difficulty with finding the voice in the noise and discriminating words correctly that were said, or in maintaining auditory attention for a specific period of time. These children are often unaware that they have heard a word or instruction correctly.
        ii) Difficulty storing and recalling auditory information in memory. These children tend to focus on and remember only part of what they heard.
        iii) Difficulty decoding and interpretating words or sounds heard in an accurate and quick manner. (Slow in figuring out words). Appeared able to decode one segment at a time and easily overloaded by lengthy information. He may

HIGH-FUNCTIONING AUTISM

show difficulty interpreting messages and language beyond the literal surface meaning and may have problems with implied meaning, multiple meaning, and inferences. He seemed often the ability to repeat back what he heard but could not interpret it completely.

iv) Had difficulty organizing and sequencing information heard, including sounds and words, words with phrases, and sentence and ideas.

In December 1987, I was given *the Wechsler Intelligence Scale for Children – Revised (WISC-R)* that resulted in a verbal IQ of 102, performance of 114 and full scale of 108.

Two months later, at, age seven years, four months old, I went to an occupational therapy (OT) screening on February 19, 1988. On the diagnosis section of the OT report it states LD, which means learning disability. The repo stated that I was referred to OT in the view of his teacher due to an observation in the classroom that showed signs of short attention span, impulsiveness, difficulty with direction and distractibility.

The OT screening method the OTR/L used was review of record, observation, demonstration of various developmental tasks, including fine-motor, gross-motor and visual-perception.

Behavioral observation on the OT report stated he was very friendly and uninhabited. Required almost constant call back on tasks. Attempted to begin tasks before instructions were completed. Quite distracted by the resource room, wanted to touch or play with everything within reasonable touch. Seemed very inquisitive. Was cooperative when tasks were sufficiently structured.

Musculoskeletal observation on the OT report stated he had normal range of motion and strength in arms. Grasp was strong in both hands. Had great difficulty in balancing on either the left or right foot. Demonstrated difficulty with reflex integration, being unable to maintain balance or show a prospective response when challenged in a "curled up" seated position. Fine-motor skills were less difficult and was able to demonstrate pinch, grasp, spontaneous release, transfer of object from hand-to-hand and opposition, and was left hand dominant.

Visual perceptual skills on the OT report stated he was able to identify left and right. Copy figures such as a Square, Triangle, Circle and the Letter X with little difficulty. He was able to draw all body parts of a human, but the figure was noticeably imbalanced. He was able to do matching tasks, but he encountered difficulty in organization, pointing to an observation that it could been connected to short attention span.

The summary of the OT report stated Mr. Boyer, age seven years, four months old, demonstrated difficulty in most areas of observation. Therefore, emphasis should be focus on improving attention span, gross motor development, future evaluation on fine-motor skills and OT should be on a regular basis.

After first grade was completed, the observation from my teacher, was summarized, and it was officially stated in the upcoming full evaluation screening and report. My teacher had "concerns about language, articulation, attention, and gross and fine motor skills" that included "numerus articulation errors, and leaves words out in sentences when speaking and writing." In addition to these issues, I had "difficulty listening to class instruction and waiting his turn." With my overall motor skills, my teacher believed they were delayed. I also suffered in "academic performance within the classroom" and it "was very inconsistent, especially in reading, arithmetic and my ability to follow instructions." Due to concerns early in the school year from my teacher, I received OT twice a month and speech and language pathology lessons four times per week at school, concentrating on auditory processing abilities.

HIGH-FUNCTIONING AUTISM

With all the testing and evaluations screening from the school year of first grade, I qualified for Learning Disability services within the school system. I received LD resources 30 to 45 minutes, three times per week due to my cognitive abilities, and the levels of achievement that were focused on my past language and auditory processing evaluations, which revealed problems in the areas of visual motor skills, auditory processing, and attention.

At the end of the first grade, my stepfather and mother described me as a boy that had difficulty comprehending (looked quite confused) while listening to stories and had difficulty with too many tasks or information overload, including interrupting many times by asking, "100's of questions," frequently. In addition, due to not keeping my hands to myself it caused self-harm such as burning my hand on a hot casserole dish. My parents questioned my judgement and worried about my unpredictable behavior and actions. My parents also stated that I was always on the go, and rarely sat down. When I was sitting down, I would fall asleep frequently a majority of the time. When in the classroom setting, I seemed to panic when no other children were around me – it was like I needed not to be alone. Other reports from my parents were getting lack of attention from me, and they would grab my chin to get me to concentrate on them when giving direction and commands they wanted me to do. At many times, my parents said I was extremely persistent in what I wanted to do and would not take "no" for an answer. More importantly, if they planned activities or tasks too far ahead, I would have an obsessive like reaction over it and worry extremely about those future tasks.

In the classroom during the first grade, it was reported from my teacher that I was always sleepy, yawning and frequently falling asleep in class and could not function after 11:30 a.m. in the classroom setting.

HIGH-FUNCTIONING AUTISM

In the home setting, I would always fall asleep during family-like meetings in the evening time with my siblings, causing my mother to think that this drowsy pattern of behavior was due to the auditory processing problems as a result of extreme level of stimuli I was getting, which overloaded me on a daily basis.

Frequented with sleep walking in the home setting, I would roam the hallways and once tried to open the back door of the home. When approached by my parents during these episodes, there was no response from me.

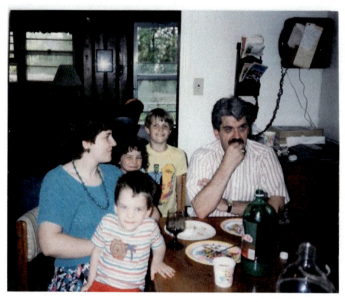

Late April 1988. Seresa's 5th Birthday Party. With Debbie Poteat, Skyler Poteat (boy), Phillip Poteat and Robert.

HIGH-FUNCTIONING AUTISM

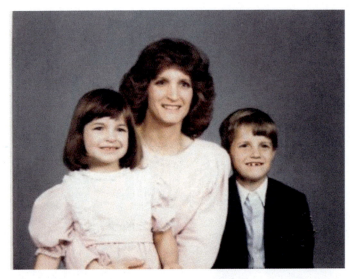

Above: 1988. Olan Mills ® photograph of Seresa, Teresa, and Robert.

Below: Mid-October of 1988. At Putt-Putt ® miniature golf located in east Burlington, North Carolina for a double Birthday Party for Robert (10/1980) and Skyler (10/1985). Their Birthdays are on October 16th.

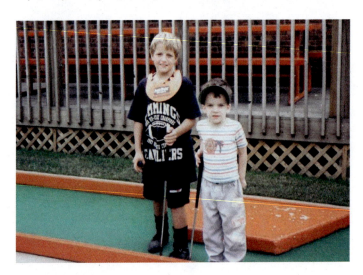

HIGH-FUNCTIONING AUTISM

On July 1, 1988, I was age seven, eight months old when I went to the Clinical Center for The Study of Development and Learning. This clinical center was part of the Child Development Research Institute of University of North Carolina at Chapel Hill (UNC-CH).

At the time of the Clinical Center evaluation, I lived with my mother, stepfather, and five-year-old baby sister. Three weeks prior to this evaluation, my mother and stepfather got married after dating for about a year. From a previous marriage, my stepfather has two daughters that spent every Wednesday evening and every other weekend with the Gentry family in 1988. During the opposite weekends, my sister and myself would visit and stay with our biological father.

During one section of the evaluation at the UNC-CH clinical center, my stepfather and mother was observing my neurological screening through a two-way mirror in the observation room. When the examiner showed my parents through the two-way mirror, my behavior shifted negatively. I screamed and yelled, saying it, "was not fair." When my parents came inside the exam room, I was comforted by my parents, and at first, I seemed content, but when I knew that my parents were going to observe me more in the observation room, I was distressed. I wanted my mother. When my parents left the exam room to continue the evaluation tasks, for a moment, the examiner got my enthusiastic in a game of "concentration," but I began to act aggressive, "in a silly manner, slamming down the cards, jumping around" and "often had trouble waiting [my] turn and had difficulty holding [my] cards." During the next task called projective testing, I continued to have negative behavioral issues. I "refused to look at any of the pictures" that were shown to me. The examiner gave me two pictures and asked to choose between the two pictures, but I said I did not like either of them. I continued to refuse the examiner's commands and only wanted my mother. I got on the exam table and jumped on it, walked on it, tried to leave the room, and then crawled under the table refusing to come out of the underbelly of the table. When the examiner was trying to get me out, I replied, "I don't like to talk!"

When the full clinic evaluation at UNC-CH was completed, the report summarized with impressions about me. It stated that I was a healthy seven-year, nine month old young boy that appeared to have attention issues and was diagnosed with deficit disorder (ADD) with characteristics of "highly impulsive, distractable, unaware of danger, very active and had great difficulties coping with transitions." Overall, my development issues were immature for my age. The high level of interference from ADD makes it difficult to confirm my degree of auditory processing problems. ADD and auditory processing are "inherently integrated and therefore will require repeated observations to clarify this issue." In addition, it was believed there was an emotional component involved with my classroom and home behavior environmental settings based on my parents' divorce, extreme sleepiness issues and the emotional lability and oppositional behavior I displayed during the clinic evaluation.

The pediatrician and registered nurse impressions on the report at UNC-CH stated that I had many characteristics of ADD. My attention weakness was more evident on tasks involving auditory input. With a previous test, it was likely I had some degree of central auditory processing disorder (CAPD/APD) in addition to my attention span issues. However, there was no clear etiology of my learning disability. My head injury at three-years-old had not placed any major concerns or pro-longed injury. With my short stature and unusual hands, it is suggested that I may have brachydactyly syndrome. There were minor neurological indicators and relative weaknesses of fine and gross motor function, which are common in a setting of a learning disability or problems in children. I had many of the behavioral

HIGH-FUNCTIONING AUTISM

manifestations of children with ADD, but it is possible that my intense reactions and my defiant behavior may reflect on some underlying emotional adjustment problems. Overall, I was a healthy child, who was seven and a half years old at the time.

After the overall evaluation in the summer of 1988, I was prescribed Ritalin for ADD – the first medication I had ever needed for any long term use for any conditions at that point in my life. I took 10 mg twice a day during the classroom and home setting.

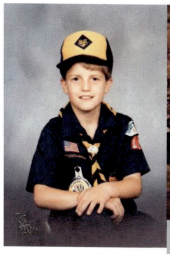

Top Left: Olan Mills ® photograph of Robert, 1989, age nine.

Top Right: Olan Mills ® photograph of Robert, 1990, age 10.

Bottom Right: Robert in 1990, age 10.

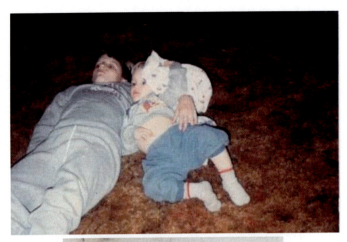

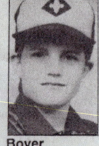

Arrow of Light

Bobby Boyer, 11, of Troop 182 at the Church of Jesus Christ of Latter Day Saints, Elon College, received the Arrow of Light Award Jan. 29 at the church.

The son of Michael Boyer and Teresa Gentry of Sherwood Drive, Burlington, Boyer has been in Scouting three years, was a denner, earned the Faith in God Award, Terrific Kid Award and placed second in Regatta, boat racing.

Boyer

Top: Robert with half-brother Jared Gentry, who was born on January 9, 1990, sometime late 1990.

Newspaper clipping in January 1992, age 11.

CHAPTER 2
MIDDLE AND HIGH SCHOOL

In 1992, with only a few weeks left in elementary school at Hillcrest, my stepfather and mother moved the family to finish out the year at Gibsonville Elementary. That school was in the Guilford County boundary of Gibsonville, which meant not only a new school but a different school system. Starting in the spring of 1992, I attended McLeansville Middle School in McLeansville.

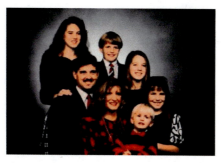

Late 1992: Olan Mills ® photograph with James Gentry (step-father) and his two children Jocelyn (behind James) and Morgan (front of Robert), from his previous marriage, including Teresa Gentry and their son, Jared and her other children, Robert, and Seresa from her previous marriage to "Mike" Boyer.

My memory is clearer, as I look back at the start of middle school. I had those narrow thoughts and had the tendency to become obsessed about topics and statistics. I was all about sports, airplanes, NASCAR, movies, and music. I *really* could drive people nuts, at times, with all the knowledge I knew, which goes back to Doctor Asperger's, "little professors," and how his patients had great knowledge and narrow, obsessive-like interests.

Hobbies that I loved to explore back in middle school included going to NASCAR weekly series races at ACE Speedway on Friday nights with my grandfather, "Marshall" Bryant and going fishing and hunting with him. Other interests I had were going camping with the Boy Scouts and going to the dances during my youth church program. I was usually too shy to dance with girls for the most part. It really took a lot of nerve to ask them to dance.

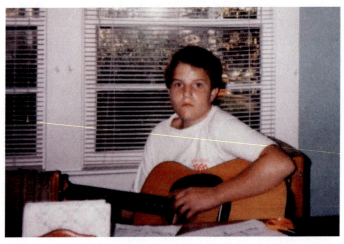

Sometime in 1992. Robert practicing guitar that was restrung for his left-handed dominant hand.

Back in the mid-1990s, I was *really* into NASCAR driver Jeff Gordon and was his biggest fan, and I collected items related to Gordon. He would become a Four-Time NASCAR Cup Series Champion over the span of his NASCAR career. I also kept tabs on a lot of the other Cup Series drivers such as Richard Petty and Dale Earnhardt, Sr. as they were tied with Seven NASCAR Cup Series Championships.

In February of 1994, I was re-evaluated for (Learning Disability) LD issues with a Verbal IQ of 80, Performance IQ of 95 and a full IQ of 86 on the *WISC-III*. My achievement standard scores on the *WJ-R* were 82 in Reading, 87 in Math and 74 in Written Language. Therefore, I was again certified as eligible for LD services, but I had not required OT or Speech/Language services.

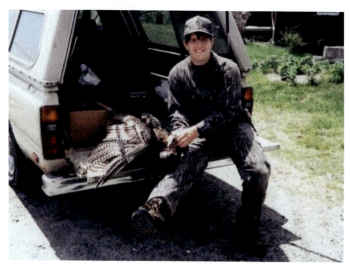

Circa 1994. First turkey Robert killed in Caswell County, North Carolina.

Here is a turkey hunting memory with my grandfather on a sunny spring morning in the mid-1990s. I think it may have been in 1994, when I was 13 years old. I killed my first turkey that was called a "Jake," an immature male. What is important and really funny about this first turkey kill was the fact that I fell asleep in the blind. I had just enough time to wake up and see the turkey poking out of the edge of the woods. It was heading out to the open field. I did not know if the turkey was a male or female due to brush being in the way but had the 12-gauge shotgun pointed and aimed at the turkey. Once I knew it was a male, I pulled the trigger. I screamed with joy, but I noticed the turkey was flopping around, so I got close to it and shot it again, which at the time I did not know the flopping was part of the turkey dying. All at the same time, my grandfather, who was hunting down the dirt road, thought I had shot myself due to the yelling and screaming of excitement as my grandfather approached my hunting area.

The first deer that I killed was during a hunt associated with my maternal great-uncle, Herbert Stainback (the brother of Hilda Marie Bryant). Even though my grandfather was not in the area where I killed my deer, which was a first-year male called a "button-head," my grandfather was close enough to see the dogs jump the herd of deer that morning in 1994.

Another thing I took up as a hobby was guitar lessons for a few years. Due to my problems with fine motor skills, it was difficult for me, but I loved to create melodies as a left-handed guitarist. After a few years of lessons, I stopped and pursued other interests in my life, such as the love of movies and getting more focused on NASCAR as I was influenced by my maternal grandfather's interest in stockcar racing.

In seventh grade and eighth grade, I was in middle school chorus, traveling to Disney World in eighth grade, which happened to be the same week of the Oklahoma City Bombing. This domestic terrorism bombing happened on April 19, 1995. The middle school chorus was part of a competition with other choruses around the nation. I remember going to the hotel room after a day at Disney World with my mother who came on the trip. She was responsible for a handful of teenage boys, including myself that was part of the chorus group during the period of the trip. Everyone turned to the TV and saw those images of the bombed federal building known as the Alfred P. Murrah Federal Building. All I can remember was the children that were in the day care, who were inside the building, that died from the act of terrorism, including the adults inside the building. It was heartbreaking.

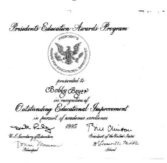

In 1995. Robert receives the President's Education Awards Program in the recognition of Outstanding Educational Improvement in pursuit of academic excellence.

During middle school I achieved some success in my academic life. At the end of eight grade, I received the *President's Education Awards Program* in the recognition of Outstanding Educational Improvement in pursuit of academic excellence, which was in 1995, and later I would receive another one in 1999 as a senior in high school.

Transitioning from McLeansville Middle School to Eastern Guilford High School in the fall of 1995 was starting to be a challenge for myself. I started to have more social deficiencies and was being bullied. I can remember getting jumped in the bathroom at least once by an upper classman while I was a freshman in high school when I was using the urinal. There were other types of bullying throughout high school that I dealt with too. I started to gain weight as well possibly from the amount of bullying, undiagnosed autism-behaviors, and my long-term "picky" diet behavior. I really did not have any friends at that moment in school, except for a few students that had similar issues of Learning Disabilities, but they were more "buddies" or acquaintances not really "true" friends. I was in special education classes as a freshman with Mrs. Cherry and later Coach Brady. With some education success in the 1995-96 school year, I lettered for academic success in 1996, at the end of my first year of high school. However, the start of the 10th grade to the end of high school, my deficiencies in language and math caused some issues in some subjects. In addition, I started to wear glasses at the end of 1996.

In 10th grade, I became one of the JV men's basketball managers for the 1996-97 season. I felt like a team player with those players and coaches because everyone had the same goals to achieve as a team not as a single person.

Due to my ongoing learning disability issues, I was sent for another psychological evaluation on January 1, 1997 at 16 years of age, due to a re-evaluation to determine my current intellectual functioning.

The re-evaluation methods used in the 1997 evaluation were the *Wechsler-Intelligence Scale for Children – Third Edition*, *Woodcock-Johnson Test of Achievement – Revised*, and *Bender Gestalt*, which at that time I was wearing my glasses and taking Ritalin.

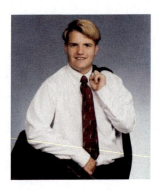

October 1996: Olan Mills ® photograph of Robert for his 16th Birthday.

HIGH-FUNCTIONING AUTISM

The psychologist stated on the 1997 evaluation notes that I was "a friendly, cooperative adolescent who was familiar with the testing procedures from previous evaluations. [I] was well aware of his LD and ADD status and volunteered that [I] hoped to attend college with the help of a scholarship for LD students. [My] attention was good throughout the testing procedures and [I] did not demonstrate any significant impulsivity. In fact, [I] was quite persistent in [my] efforts, and often would work very hard on tasks in trying to reach a solution. [My] speech was easily understood, and [my] verbal responses were appropriate. However, [I] commented several times on the Vocabulary subtest of the *WISC-III* that [I] knew the word's meaning, but just could not find a way to explain it. The current test results are felt to be an accurate reflection of [my] intellectual functioning." The test results of *WISC-III* IQs were the following: 93 on Verbal, 95 on Performance, and 93 on Full Scale.

The summary section of the 1997 evaluation, which highlights some red flags of high-functioning autism, which states that I was "friendly, cooperative adolescent who is currently functioning in the Average range of intelligence. There was no significant discrepancy between Verbal and Performance IQs, but [my] Verbal IQ [had] increased significantly since the previous evaluation. Nevertheless, [I continued] to manifest a deficit in [my] expressive vocabulary. [My] visual-motor integration [was] within Average range, as [were my] overall math skills. [My] reading and written language skills [were] in the Low Average range."

Throughout the 11th to 12th grade, I became the Varsity Basketball Men's Manager for 11th and 12th grades, playing football in the 11th grade and was the manager in the 12th grade for the football team. My favorite subject in school was drafting, influenced by my stepfather, but I feel like I also had the artistic creativity of a drafting-like mind (and

HIGH-FUNCTIONING AUTISM

that didn't hurt). During the same period, I struggled in advanced math, some science classes like chemistry (I failed), English and Spanish classes.

On April 1, 1999, for the second time in my life, I went back to the UNC-CH Clinic Center that I first went to in 1988. The reason why I went back to the clinic was due to my continued weight gain, which I "reported significant problems with settling to sleep and awakening once or more nightly." It was reported that I was a "bad snorer" and there was no observation if I stopped breathing for a period of time, but I stated that I had jerking in my legs and had restless sleep.

In the development history of the updated 1999 UNC-CH Clinic Center it stated that I had some good friends at the same time of my weight gain between 9th and 10th grade. At that point of my life, my mother stated, based on the report notes, that "Adults were his friends." I told the healthcare team at the clinic that "Teasing has been going on as long as I can remember…At least since the seventh grade…I talk slow…they say I talk like Forrest Gump." To deflect the bullying, I would laugh and joke it off. My interest in sports led me to manage the sports teams in high school. However, it did not help my social awkwardness to make friends, despite being part of the sports teams in high school. Therefore, I would spend much of my social time alone in my bedroom or computer room playing computer games and watching TV.

My behavioral issues that are stated in the 1999 UNC-CH Clinic Center documentation states that I had "been depressed" since my weight gain. I do not really get too mad, but when it does happen, I storm around, slam doors and throw things. I had never seen a counselor but was comfortable talking to my mother about my issues. However, I never discussed my issues about the bullying I had suffered in middle and high school. It was reported that my parents were not aware of any family members that showed any intellectual disabilities or any other serious learning problems, genetic disorders, obesity issues or autism previously. Therefore, the previous diagnosis from the prior visit in 1988 was now upgraded to the Adult form of ADD, but due to the lack of knowledge of what was still called Asperger's syndrome (officially high-functioning autism, as of 2013), the healthcare team at UNC-CH Clinic Center allegedly misdiagnosed or underdiagnosed me for not having any form of autism.

My first NASCAR Cup Series race (known as the Winston Cup Series in 1999) was at Martinsville Speedway with my maternal grandparents, Marshall and Hilda and sister, Seresa. It was the first time I experienced the smells, noise, and the excitement of what I was missing in stockcar racing. I had only a glimpse of it in the amateur racing series at ACE Speedway, but that first race at an actual Cup Series event was a big eye opener and it set the path for a multitude of in-person races to cheer on my favorite, Jeff Gordon.

Senior Night Awards, near the end of the graduating school year, was in late May of 1999. I received Draftsman of the Year in my drafting class.

During my graduation rehearsal inside the school's cafeteria, a classmate pulled a chair out from beneath me, as I was getting ready to sit down, causing myself to fall hard onto the solid floor. I ran out of the cafeteria immediately due to the *major* embarrassment. That student should not have walked on graduation day for that bullying behavior, but he did. My mother and I were puzzled why he was allowed to walk after what he did. We felt that it was just ridiculous that he was not held accountable for his actions. My mother was very upset that there were no other disciplinary actions for the aggressor's bullying behavior. In fact, I was not only embarrassed, but I could have gotten seriously injured from the fall to onto the hard floor.

When I graduated from Eastern Guilford High School

in 1999, my final GPA was 2.536, and I was ranked 69 of 149 graduating seniors, putting me at 46.3% of the overall graduating class.

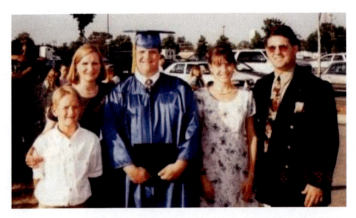

Above: June 13, 1999. EGHS Graduation. Left to Right Jared, Teresa, Robert, Seresa, and James.

Below: Summer 1998. Horseback riding in Tennessee Mountains during a family vacation.

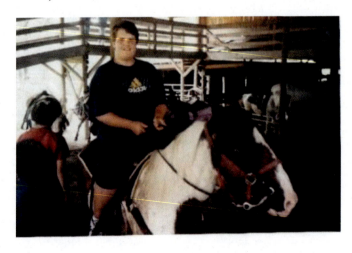

HIGH-FUNCTIONING AUTISM

President's Education Awards Program

presented to
Robert Boyer
in recognition of
Outstanding Educational Improvement
in pursuit of academic excellence

Dick Riley — 1999 — Bill Clinton
U.S. Secretary of Education — President of the United States

Linda Maler — Eastern Guilford High
Principal — School

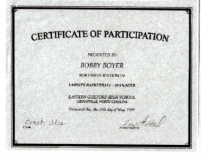

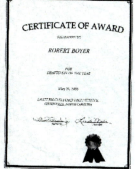

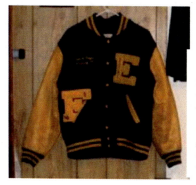

Eastern Guilford High School "Letter Jacket" with a 1996 Academic Letter in Ninth Grade, additional letter for playing football in 11th Grade, and two gold medal pins for football and basketball managers during 11th and 12th Grades.

HIGH-FUNCTIONING AUTISM

CHAPTER 3
SUMMER 1999 TO SUMMER 2002

    A new chapter started after high school graduation from Eastern Guilford High School. We set out in our family van on an adventure out west to Utah. The trip took us to Graceland to see Elvis's home and museum, Oklahoma City to see the 1995 Oklahoma City Bombing location, Grand Canyon, a brief trip to see Las Vegas with my stepfather's sister and some of her children's families that lived in the southern Utah city of St. George and central Utah Salt Lake City valley, and northern Utah, and Yellowstone Park. After leaving Utah, my family went to the Snake River, Great Plains and St. Louis. In all, this was a very, action packed, two-week trip that happened in the summer of 1999. Our goal was to visit the historic sites of The Church of Jesus Christ of Latter-day Saints and to see family from my stepfather and mother's side of the family.

    After getting back from the trip, sometime in late June or July of 1999, I began working as a bagger for Food Lion. That job was difficult for the nearly 12 months of working due to my limitations. I struggled with the fast pace of keeping up with bagging items for the customers. My other duties included cleaning up spills, cleaning the restrooms, cleaning the floors and some stocking during less busy times during my shift.

HIGH-FUNCTIONING AUTISM

During the 12 months at Food Lion, I was also in the midst of planning for my volunteer church mission for The Church of Jesus Christ of Latter-day Saints (Church), which would be a full-time mission for two years. There were a multitude of delays due to figuring out what was best for me. There was additional counseling that was provided to figure out my mental and emotional state due to some medications I was taking at the time for my learning disability and ADHD issues.

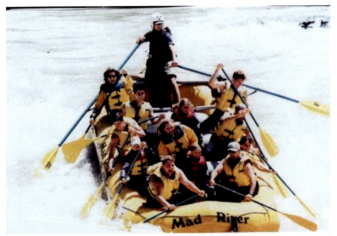

Summer of 1999 on the Snake River at Jackson, Wyoming. Bottom left corner is Robert, Jared (center front), James (bottom right), Seresa (behind James) and Teresa (behind Jared) during a white-water rafting event during the cross-country family trip.

During the delay in trying to figure out about serving a full-time, two-year mission, I was able to go through the open house and dedication of the North Carolina Raleigh Temple of the Church in late 1999.

Starting in 2000, I had to go to counseling for the first time. It was to see if I was mentally fit to serve a two-year, full-time mission for the Church. I had a few sessions with a counselor with a Master's degree in science, and with the first session I was diagnosed with depression, but not clinically depressed at that point. I had to go through all the counseling sessions that were required by the Church in order to qualify to serve my mission. My counselor was a member of the Church's Family Services department of the global wide LDS Church.

Finally, in the middle of 2000, I got the official letter that I would be serving a mission for the Church. I was originally assigned to the Des Moines Iowa Mission. I would report to the Mission Training Center (MTC) in Provo, Utah in August 2000.

Before reporting to the MTC, I had to complete vaccinations, get my wisdom teeth removed, purchase clothing such as dress suits, ties, shirts, and shoes. Since it was in the Midwest where I was going to serve, I also needed some winter clothing and had to have a bicycle for my mission to ride with my companions when not using a mission-owned car. In addition, I would have to go through the temple myself for a special service called an Endowment (a special blessing and ceremony) for worthy men and women of the Church before they start a mission or other qualifying events.

In August 2002, my maternal grandparents went with me to Utah to send me off to the MTC to start my mission for the Church. Back before September 11, 2001, anyone could go to the gates to send off people before they were ready to board the airplane. That was my experience in August 2002.

In Utah, my grandparents and I stayed with some family members from my maternal grandmother's side of her family called the Ouzts Family. They lived outside of Salt Lake City. Even my mother stayed with this family sometimes when she was attending the Church-owned Brigham Young University (BYU) in the late 1970s. During the brief family trip before entering the MTC, I went through the Salt Lake Temple with my grandparents and visited other church sites around Temple Square, like the Visitor Center of Temple Square.

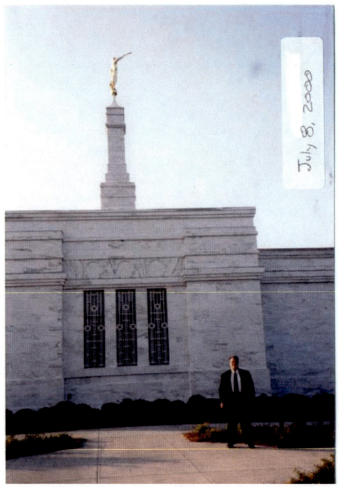

July 8, 2000. Robert in front of the Raleigh North Carolina Temple (The Church of Jesus Christ of Latter-day Saints). One month before the church mission.

HIGH-FUNCTIONING AUTISM

During the Farewell meeting inside the MTC, my grandparents and I said our goodbyes and I started a three-week training at the MTC to enter the mission field in Iowa.

Inside the MTC, it was a college-like setting where hundreds of missionaries were training and learning the material to prepare to become a missionary for the Church.

I became Elder Boyer for two years, after getting set apart (ordained) as a full-time volunteer missionary back in North Carolina by my Stake President. The Stake President is over at least 10 to 12 congregations that are called Branches or Wards in a regional geographical area. At that time, I was part of the Durham Stake that covered Durham, Chapel Hill, Henderson, South Boston (Virginia), Roxboro and Burlington congregations. Some cities had more than one congregation that were in the same chapel or separate chapel.

While at the MTC, I got sick and I could not do some of the activities. However, my experience was fun with my MTC companion. I stayed in my dorm room for a few days when sick. Inside the MTC dorm room, there were two sets of bunkbeds for the missionaries to sleep in.

A day as a MTC missionary was to get up around six in the morning, having personal and companionship study, get a shower, eat breakfast, and go to classes. Then after lunch go to more classes. One day of the week would be a preparation day like washing clothing, writing home to family and friends, physical activities like sports and personal time. This type of schedule would continue into the mission field, but instead of classes, the missionaries would knock on doors, get media and family referrals to teach the Missionary Discussions to those who wanted to learn and become members of the Church. In addition, in the mission field, each assigned area had four hours of community service duties a week such as working at libraries, food kitchens, community zoos and other types of volunteer opportunities based on resources available in the assigned areas.

HIGH-FUNCTIONING AUTISM

In the MTC, it was hard memorizing the Missionary Discussions due to my LD and ADD issues, but I had a great spirit, and many others around me saw that quality. Members of the Church and community where I served were touched about how my personality was a blessing in their lives. Overall, my communication and social skills improved as a missionary, but there were, and will always be, deficits in these areas of my personality.

Once in the first area of my mission, I was informed that the area Church congregations that are known as a Ward or Branch inside one Stake of the Church were transferring from the Iowa Des Moines Mission to the Illinois Peoria Mission geographical boundaries, starting in early November 2000. The Stake being transferred over was the Davenport Stake in Iowa, which covered both Iowa and Illinois congregations along the Mississippi River area.

Not even a month into the church mission in Clinton, Iowa, I ended up sick and had to go to the doctor, who was also a member of the Church. I was diagnosed with a sinus infection, high blood pressure, and morbid obesity on September 9, 2000. I ended up on Medications including Vasotec for my blood pressure and antibiotics for my sinus infection.

Three weeks later for a follow-up, in September 2000, with the Clinton doctor, the diagnoses included ADHD, high blood pressure and depression. My weight jumped up a few more pounds to 271 from the previous visit. Medications included Ritalin (for ADHD), Wellbutrin (for depression) and to continue the Vasotec (for high blood pressure), Also the doctor added Celexa for Depression and ADHD.

Not even two weeks later, I was seen on September 29, 2000 for a "Flu-like" illness. My vital signs were pretty much the same, but my weight dropped from 271 to 267 pounds (-4 lbs). My treatment plan was treating the Flu-like illness.

HIGH-FUNCTIONING AUTISM

In early November 2000, about 24 missionaries, including myself, were transferred into the new mission called Illinois Peoria Mission, which included the Nauvoo area, which the Nauvoo Temple was getting re-built, nearly a duplication of the original that was abandoned and torn down by a fire, and later by a tornado back in the mid-1800s when the Church Pioneers were driven out of Illinois by anti-Mormon mobs, and the Pioneers finally moved to Salt Lake City.

That same week, when the mission boundaries were changed, the missionaries were invited to the Symbolic Cornerstone Ceremony at the Nauvoo Temple on November 5, 2000 that included the late President Gordon B. Hinckley who was over the global church along with general and area representatives of the Church.

It was December 26, 2000 when I was really sick. Very nauseous and vomiting. The next day I went to see the Clinton doctor. At the December 27, 2000 doctor's appointment, I was diagnosed with flu-like illness and treated as such with the proper medications. My vitals were the same and I lost one pound with a weight of 270. However, only a few days later, on January 4, 2001, I was worse off with the flu-like illness and gained six pounds with a weight of 276.

Between January 2001 to July 12, 2001, I started to have issues that would be diagnosed as an Anal Fissure and my weight jumped to 285. Riding the bike flared this issue up over the span of months. The pain of having anal issues and painful bowel movements from the torn anal muscle caused much stress.

A follow-up visit on July 24, 2001 showed more issues, including internal hemorrhoids. The next appointment, which was associated with the anal fissure was August 21, 2001. There was blood in my stool sample, and I was in a lot of pain. My BP was a little more elevated (142/87). My blood pressure probably elevated due to the amount of pain

HIGH-FUNCTIONING AUTISM

I was in much of the time. Due to the stresses of the anal fissure, my complications of ADD and morbid obesity was addressed at the Clinton doctor's appointment dated on October 30, 2001. In the October appointment my vitals were stable as they were in my last appointment, but the BP was more stable at 133/76. Another condition started to be an issue, which was dry skin on scalp called Seborrheic dermatitis and that was addressed with the Clinton doctor on November 13, 2001 and a treatment plan was provided for that condition. At the November appointment my weight came down from the mid-280s to the weight of 278. My other vitals were stable from the previous appointment.

In a letter dated December 5, 2001, which was addressed to the vocational rehabilitation (VR) services in North Carolina (NC), the Clinton doctor wrote that he first saw me, starting on September 7, 2000, for treatment of "ADHD, hypertension, and morbid obesity" with issues of "functional disabilities" such as "auditory processing deficiencies" and "fine motor skills problems in his hands." He stated that I needed the following medications for attending college, starting in the fall of 2002, which were Celexa 20mg and Concerta 36mg daily for ADHD, Vasotec for hypertension, and Meridia for obesity. He stated while I was on the ADHD medication that "he still has some functional limitations that may limit him in the future as far as finding a well paying job."

Due to the continuing issues with the anal fissure, I was sent home in late December of 2001 or early January 2002 for surgery for an anal fissure repair. I was still set apart as a missionary for the Church, and I had the surgery and would go back on my mission in March 2002, after my recovering.

During the post-surgery and recovery, my mother and I went to Haywood Community College (HCC) so I could take some placement tests for the upcoming fall semester.

HIGH-FUNCTIONING AUTISM

We traveled to the North Carolina mountain city of Clyde where HCC is located.

The placement tests that I took, dated February 15, 2001, are below.

> i) Reading (scale range 35-80) was 60, percentile of 23.
> ii) Sentence Skills (scale range 30-86) was 59, percentile of 20.
> iii) Arithmetic (scale range 25-57) was 79, percentile of 82.
> iv) Algebra (scale range 0-60) was 41, percentile of 54.

The placement classes included RED 090, ENG 090 and MAT 070.

Once back into the mission field in Illinois, I continued to have issues with my anal fissure recovery, ADHD, and other issues previously addressed during my mission. However, I only had three months left on my mission by the time I returned in March 2002. For the remainder of my mission, I dealt with my pain and other developmental issues.

On June 26, 2002, I was released into the authority of my family that included my stepfather, mother, and my maternal grandparents. Over ten family members came out to pick me up from my mission as they traveled by vehicle. We would visit around the mission boundaries to see people that I got to know, visit historic Nauvoo and Carthage Jail, and be part of the first session of the dedication of the newly built temple inside the Nauvoo Temple on June 27, 2002, which also marked the martyrdom of Joseph Smith and his brother Hyrum, which was 158 years earlier on June

HIGH-FUNCTIONING AUTISM

27, 1844 at the location of Carthage Jail when an anti-Mormon mob busted through the jail and shot and killed the Smith brothers.

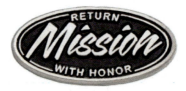

With all said and done, I learned a lot, and my developmental issues had improved, but I still had a long way to go, and was still living with the undiagnosed case of autism. Having the undiagnosed case of autism would continue to be a problem post-mission for The Church of Jesus Christ of Latter-day Saints in the Illinois Peoria Mission. However, I grew in other ways despite the limitations of my disabilities that are physical, mental, and emotional. I learned great lessons about who I was as a missionary, overall.

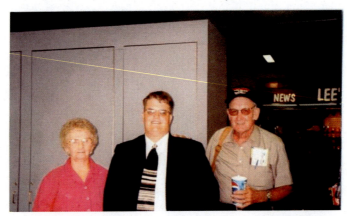

August 13, 2000 at the RDU Airport between Raleigh and Durham. Hilda Stainback Bryant, Robert, and Joseph Marshall Bryant. They traveled with their grandson to Utah to send him off on his church mission.

HIGH-FUNCTIONING AUTISM

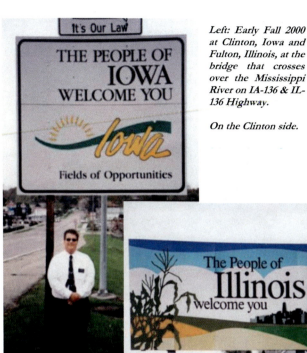

Left: Early Fall 2000 at Clinton, Iowa and Fulton, Illinois, at the bridge that crosses over the Mississippi River on IA-136 & IL-136 Highway.

On the Clinton side.

Right: Early Fall 2000 at Clinton, Iowa and Fulton, Illinois, at the bridge that crosses over the Mississippi River on IA-136 & IL-136 Highway.

On the Fulton side.

HIGH-FUNCTIONING AUTISM

NAUVOO TEMPLE
SYMBOLIC CORNERSTONE CEREMONY
November 5, 2000

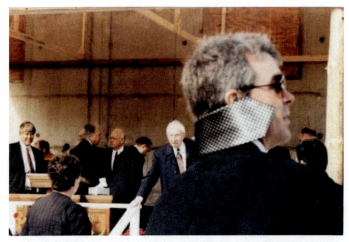

The symbolic laying of cornerstones at the Nauvoo Temple took place on Sunday, Nov. 5, 2000, at noon in Nauvoo, Ill. The late President Gordon B. Hinckley of the Church is at center on top picture.

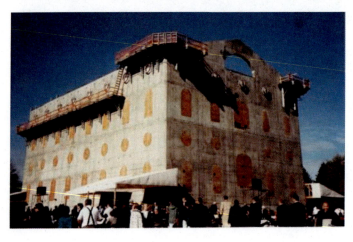

HIGH-FUNCTIONING AUTISM

NAUVOO TEMPLE CONSTRUCTION
SPRING 2001

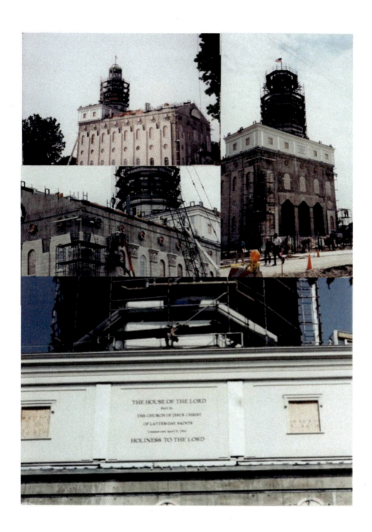

HIGH-FUNCTIONING AUTISM

NAUVOO TEMPLE CONSTRUCTION
FALL 2001 & MARCH 2002

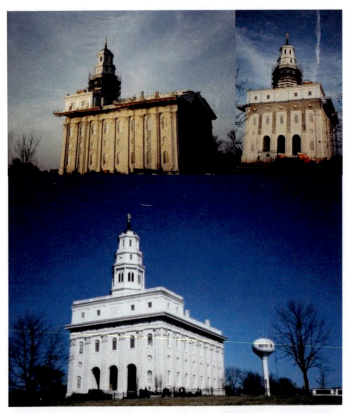

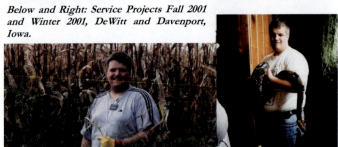

Below and Right: Service Projects Fall 2001 and Winter 2001, DeWitt and Davenport, Iowa.

HIGH-FUNCTIONING AUTISM

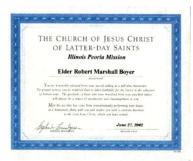

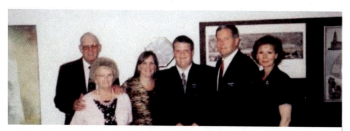

Above: June 26, 2002 in the Mission Home with President Lundgreen and Sister Lundgreen. Left to Right: "Marshall", Hilda, Teresa, Robert, President Lundgreen and Sister Lundgreen.

Below: June 26, 2002 outside the Mission Home with President Lundgreen and Sister Lundgreen. Left to Right (Front Row): President Lundgreen, Sister Lundgreen, Teresa, Kelsey Bryant, Jared, Justin Bryant, Hilda. Left to Right (Back Row): James, Maghen Bryant, Robert, Phillip Poteat, Skyler Poteat, Marshall, Allen Dwyane Bryant, and Tabby Bryant.

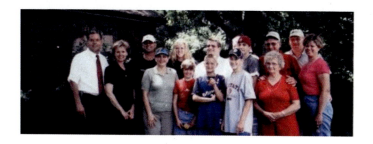

HIGH-FUNCTIONING AUTISM

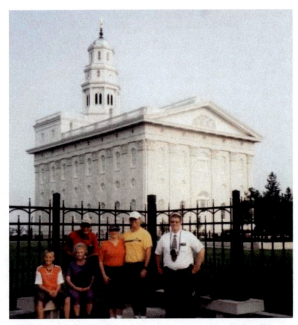

Above: June 27, 2002 at the Nauvoo Temple post-dedication ceremony. Left to Right: Jared, Hilda, Marshall, Teresa, James, and Robert.

Below: June 27, 2002 at Carthage, Illinois on horseback on the original path to Carthage Jail that Joseph Smith and Hyrum Smith took when arrested with false allegations back in 1844 before they were killed by the anti-Mormon mob. Front to Back: Kelsey, Jared, Tabby, Robert, and Dwayne.

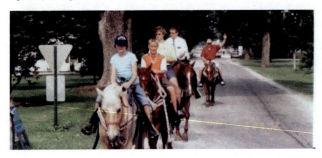

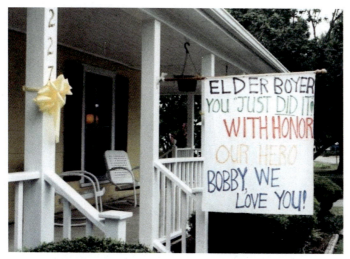

July 2002 in front of the teenage home of Robert in celebration of his return from his church mission.

Below is one of a few name tags Mr. Boyer wore on his church mission.

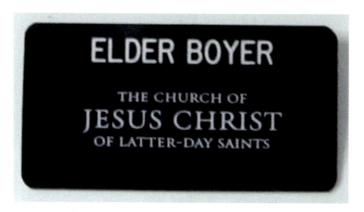

HIGH-FUNCTIONING AUTISM

HIGH-FUNCTIONING AUTISM

CHAPTER 4
JULY 2002 TO JUNE 23, 2012

A few weeks after being released as a missionary for my church, I went to the North Carolina Department of Health and Human Resources Division of Vocational Rehabilitation Services for testing on July 24, 2002. I was 21 years old at the time. The following scores from the *Woodcock-Johnson Test of Achievement (WJ-III)* regarding Learning Disability services are below and are believed valid.

(a) Broad Reading, which contains the following issues of Letter-Word Identification, Reading Fluency and Passage Comprehension was a Grade Equivalent of 6.3.
(b) Written Expression, which contains the following issues of Writing Fluency and Writing Sample was a Grade Equivalent of 6.7.

I was given assistance from VR to attend Haywood Community College for Wildlife Management, but due to the struggles of learning scientific-like studies in the association of Wildlife Management, I would switch from that course of study to Film and Video Production Technology the following year. I ended up having to take placement classes at HCC over the next two semesters, failing Algebra once in the fall semester. However, I passed Algebra in the spring semester. Throughout the one year at HCC, I never had any friends. The 7-studio apartment complex, which I lived in, was across the campus. There were students in the Wildlife Program, but they were not the type of students I really clicked with. I did socialize with them, tried to be a friendly guy, but other than that, I just stayed clear from them. I would stay in my studio apartment and study and would write on my spare time. I worked on a superhero novel. I would go to movies occasionally. At the time I drove a green extended cab S-10 Chevrolet 4x4 pickup truck, which I had to use in the winter of 2002-2003 due to the snow in the mountains. I would also go to see the Elk, which were at the nearby Great Smoky Mountains National Park where they were introduced into the Chattahoochee Valley in 2001 and 2002.

The Chattahoochee Valley once was private land, but the federal government bought the land, and the government restored and preserved the historic buildings in the valley that include two churches, a school and several homes and outbuildings. There are also gravesites in the valley from the late 19th to early 20th Century eras. The only way to get to the area is by a few narrow, curvy mountain roads that are mostly gravel.

I enjoyed the valley where I could look for elk and other wildlife in the area. It was a peaceful place to get away from the worries of the world, including my personal struggles of my undiagnosed autism and other developmental and mental issues, which effected my mental, emotional, medical, and physical issues.

HIGH-FUNCTIONING AUTISM

In the summer of 2003, my father visited me. Also, I took some film classes at HCC as I transferred my Associate's Degree to Film and Video Production Technology, which I would transfer to Piedmont Community College – Caswell Campus in the Fall of 2003, living with my maternal grandparents during the week since the community college was 10 miles from their home that is located in southern Caswell County.

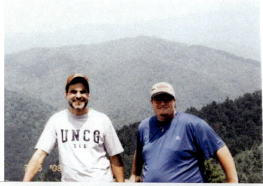

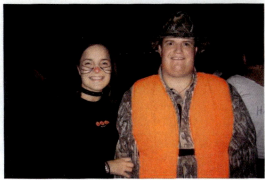

Above: 2003. Haywood County, North Carolina. Robert with his father Mike.

Below. Halloween Party 2002. Robert with his sister Seresa

HIGH-FUNCTIONING AUTISM

The start of the film program studies was a blessing for me. I found my niche in life, which I had at least a decade of having a narrow, obsessive-like following for the topics of film. I especially loved the film *Titanic* from 1997 that was written and directed by James Cameron. I saw this film in the theater about half a dozen times. I was not alone, a lot of people were with me, watching it over and over. Other genres of films that I continue to love are war movies, action movies, superhero movies and movies based on true events.

During the course of the film program at PCC-Caswell Campus, I was required to attend film productions within the program, which were short films. There were at least three films, included was a music video. The music video was edited by students and the band liked my concept of the edited music video that I did. The simple editing concept was my love on top of filming. I had always loved making home movies but could not edit them. I just loved to film anything when I had a chance to.

During my last year of obtaining my Associate's Degree, at the end of the year awards, I won the Outstanding Student of the program and I had a GPA of 3.50. I was not on any medication for ADHD or LD issues, other than for high blood pressure, I do recall.

Before graduating from PCC, I tried to get into local news stations, as far as Charlotte, North Carolina, but those plans on getting a job in a relevant field of study never happened for me. It was a personal blow to my mental state of mind, but it really goes back to my ADHD, LD, and the undiagnosed autism.

In May 2005, I got a third-shift security guard job that protected clients' assets throughout the Greensboro and Burlington area of North Carolina. This was a part-time job, which paid approximately eight dollars an hour in 2005. This company kept on screwing up my paychecks, paying me only half what I worked. My mother, as an advocate for me, went with me to the office of the company and tried to settle this issue, but again it never was settled. Finally, I walked off the job not knowing when I would get another job. But, I got hired soon after walking off my first job. I was hired at a local private university as a third-shift security guard protecting the football stadium area two nights a week, paying approximately seven and a half dollars an hour in late 2005.

During the time I was working as a security guard at the university, I went to the North Carolina DMV school to get a Commercial Driver's License (CDL) for driving a school bus for the public school system, which it was free. I passed the course and got the CDL Class B with passenger and school bus endorsements, but later I got the tank endorsement.

Due to getting the CDL Class B, I had a lead to get a job, but it fell through, leaving me out of the security guard job because I already quit the job, thinking I had the job related to the CDL position. However, this was never the case. It had been a misleading or miscommunication issue that put another blow into my mental state of mind in early 2006.

Things finally started to change when a local public school system hired me as a part-time school bus driver. Briefly it was substitute status for nearly two weeks. This job started in April 2006.

Training as a school bus driver – in real-life situations – on the job training was an eye opener. It was a hard job because public government officials allegedly would not handle unsafe situations from repeat aggressors in a stronger way. These issues were so unsafe, it caused me to have my first at-fault accidents in my life as a general person with a driver's license.

From the time I started working for the public school system to the time I resigned in early 2019, things changed. The student behavior was so bad that nationally there was

HIGH-FUNCTIONING AUTISM

a continuation of bus driver shortages due to what I personally experienced everyday of bullying from students against bus drivers, which in the case with me, it felt like I was attending high school all over again with all the teasing and bullying that I felt as a teenager, many years earlier.

The only reason I put up with this daily abuse was the benefits that came later in 2008 when I was full-time status. I would get health insurance, but again, due to the low pay of a bus driver, it was a catch 22. My wages were up and down each year, including a pay freeze for a few years and the highest I ever got paid was a gross of approximately $23,000, but the last few years that gross dropped to about $21,000 by the year I left in 2019.

Why suffer through the politics of trying to please the parents and the child, and your boss for that kind of pay? It's quite ridiculous actually. If a child is misbehaving, you're supposed to discipline a child while keeping the bus in control at the same time, while making all your stops within a certain amount of time. These children are not the same kids I went to school with. Some of them have absolutely no respect for authority whatsoever.

Due to the part-time status as a bus driver from 2006 to late 2008, I bought some video equipment and did take on some side gigs.

In the summer of 2006, I started to film local bands that I became friends with. But before I got my professional gear, I would use home video cameras and edit the videos together. Filming the bands, or private events like weddings, was fun, but really the time put into the projects was not worth the money. I was not paid to film the local bands because I was friends with some of them. I made music videos from their live recordings that I filmed. It was a great experience, and it channeled my creativity, and the narrow, obsessive-like topics that comes from those autism characteristics.

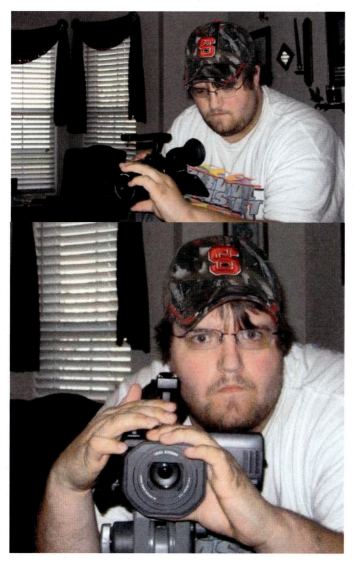

Sometime in 2008. Robert with his Panasonic Pro AG-DVC30 3-CCD MiniDV Camcorder w/16x Optical Zoom.

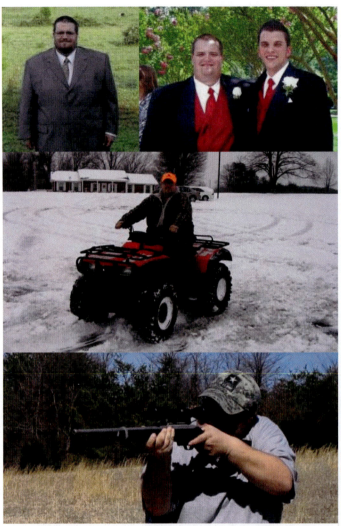

Top Left: Robert, April 2009. Top Right: Robert and Skyler, August 1, 2009 at his wedding. Center, Robert, January 31, 2010 at Caswell Ward of The Church of Jesus Christ of Latter-day Saints with his maternal grandparents' home in background. Bottom: Robert, February 2010 on the Bryant Homestead in Caswell County.

HIGH-FUNCTIONING AUTISM

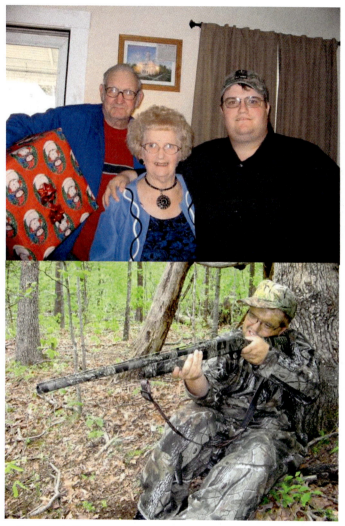

Top: March 2010 Robert with Marshall and Hilda at Robert's open house Coble Street, Burlington, NC.

Bottom: April 2011. Robert during Turkey Season.

HIGH-FUNCTIONING AUTISM

QUICK COURTSHIP AND ENGAGEMENT
Karen Melissa Ray and Robert Marshall Boyer
Met on eHarmony in mid-November 2011
Engaged December 29, 2011

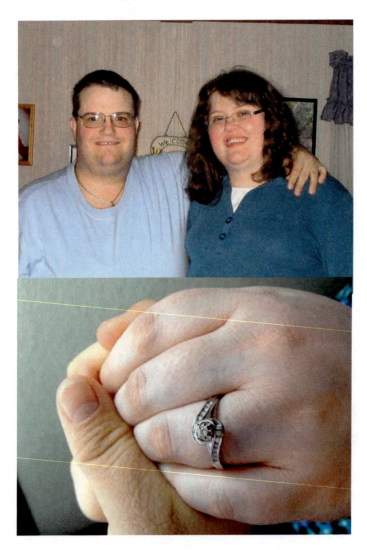

HIGH-FUNCTIONING AUTISM

ENGAGEMENT PHOTO
Karen Melissa Ray and Robert Marshall Boyer
March 31, 2012

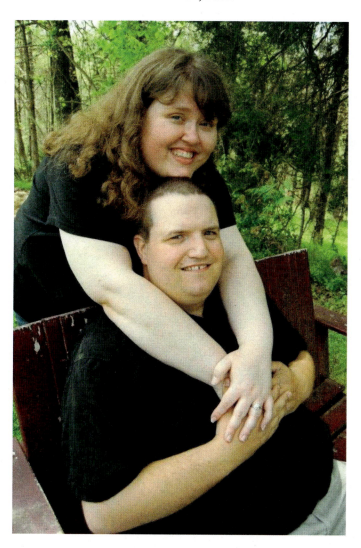

HIGH-FUNCTIONING AUTISM

WEDDING DAY
Karen Melissa Ray and Robert Marshall Boyer
Green Bank, West Virginia
June 23, 2012

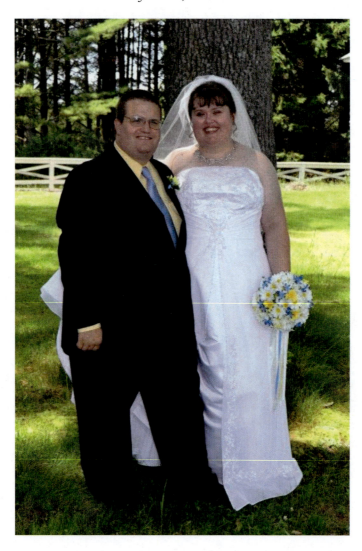

HIGH-FUNCTIONING AUTISM

WEDDING DAY
Karen Melissa Ray and Robert Marshall Boyer
Green Bank, West Virginia
June 23, 2012

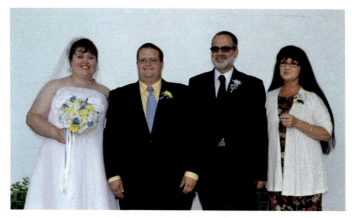

Above: Karen, Robert, Mike, and Sherry Boyer

Below: James, Karen, Robert, and Teresa Bryant.

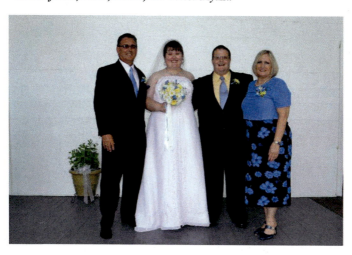

HIGH-FUNCTIONING AUTISM

WEDDING DAY
Karen Melissa Ray and Robert Marshall Boyer
Green Bank, West Virginia
June 23, 2012

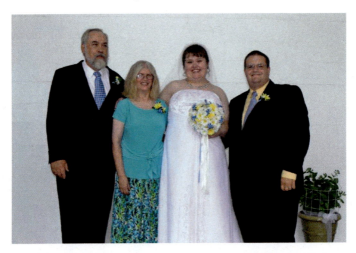

James "Jim" Ray, Kathy Ray, Karen Ray Boyer, and Robert Marshall Boyer

James Watkins Gentry, my stepfather, officiated the wedding. At the time, my stepfather was a Bishop in the Gibsonville Ward for The Church of Jesus Christ of Latter-day Saints and could officiate the wedding.

After the wedding reception, we drove to Pigeon Forge, Tennessee to Dollywood and visited a few areas surrounding Sevierville and Gatlinburg on our honeymoon.

A few weeks later, we had an open house at the Gibsonville Ward of The Church of Jesus Christ of Latter-day Saints.

My chapter had ended as a single person. My wife and I had a shared a history of several failed romantic relationships. We both ended up trying eHarmony, the science and questions matched us up. We clicked instantly when we met and immediately bonded. Karen was crying when she had to leave after the first visit. We definitely didn't have a traditional courtship and wedding.

We were independently thinking about ending our subscriptions for eHarmony in November 2019. Karen's subscription was ending sometime in November and my subscription sometime sooner. We were about to give up in finding someone to have a romantic relationship. We both had failed romantic relationships over the years, and we were in our early 30s at the time, and we were losing hope for a companion. By the time we were independently getting ready to shut down our subscriptions of the dating website, we were matched up. I believe I took the first communication steps provided by eHarmony. Then the rest was history making, which was a fast paced relationship that evolved to an engagement approximately a month later. Within the first days of getting matched up in November 2011, we visited each other for the first time when Karen traveled to North Carolina to a Christmas gathering. Karen says she was at work on break when I messaged her and mentioned the possibility of her coming to the family Christmas Party, if she was able. She was looking at her schedule and actually happened to be off the days the gathering was happening. It was like it was meant to be, as funny as that sounds. In our second visit, in late December 2011, we were engaged on December 29, 2011 when I went to Elkins, West Virginia to visit her at her home.

When shopping for the engagement ring, I told my then girlfriend Karen to see if the ring was going to fit, which it did, and I said something in the terms, "okay, it fits, and let's get married." I technically never proposed to my then fiancée, Karen Melissa Ray. If you think of it in my point of view, my brain functions were, and still are, wired to function like that. Well, it all goes back to the autism characteristics. Karen says I still owe her a proper engagement and says maybe for one of our anniversaries I can propose to her.

Once engaged, I went back to North Carolina and Karen continued to look for work for her pending move to North Carolina. It was an anxiety-inducing process. It took a little while to get the things going to get a registered nursing license in North Carolina. There were delays due to bad fingerprinting by the WV State Police. Lost Fingerprints in the US Postal System, and other protocols delayed the process. Finally, all things came together, and she got her RN license in NC to practice nursing. She landed a job as a Home Health Nurse case manager in April of 2012. At the same time that she was interviewing for the job, she did some wedding dress shopping down in NC with me, which was another non-traditional wedding thing, but that was how we started things, and that was how we rolled, I guess. I actually went to David's Bridal with her to pick out the dress. The lady helping her thought we were insane. She was like, "Uh, are you the groom. You're not supposed to see her in the dress, right?" Karen was like, "No it's fine, we're old." And laughed.

Once the perfect dress was chosen, which happened to be the very first dress she picked out and tried on, Karen was ready for getting her bridal pictures taken, which happened in Caswell County on some of my families' property on the Bryant Homestead, formally part of the Walter Stainback Farm. Mr. Stainback is my maternal grandmother's father, making me his great-grandson.

A brief story about Mr. Stainback. He was the one that unknowingly inspired Jonathan Byrd Bryant (my great grandfather) and his family to move from Carroll County, Virginia to live with them on the Stainback Farm to farm tobacco. Mr. Stainback ran a newspaper ad looking for LDS members to help farm his land. He knew that the Bryant Family was also members of the church. At that time there were very few members of the church in the eastern part of the United States and fewer in Virginia and North Carolina. This was back in the mid-1940s. Mr. Bryant responded to the newspaper ad and uprooted his family, including his only son Joseph Marshall Bryant, who was 12 years old at the time, to Caswell County, North Carolina in the Township of Anderson.

Now back to the present day. From March 2012 to June 23, 2012, we only had around 90 days to get everything ready for the wedding. Since my stepfather was an active Bishop for The Church of Jesus Christ of Latter-day Saints, I took the steps to get him set up to be able to officiate the wedding. I sent in an application and fee for the State of West Virginia. The wedding was in Green Bank, which connects to the south of Karen's home, the unincorporated town of Arbovale, WV.

Arbovale and Green Bank are located in the County of Pocahontas, West Virginia. The county is located in eastern central WV, bordering the east-central area of the State of Virginia. One of the great treasures in the area is the famous Green Bank Observatory (formally known as part of the National Radio Astronomy Observatory, until September 30, 2016). The observatory has the world's largest fully steerable radio telescope, surpassing the Effelsberg 100-m Radio Telescope in Germany. The world's largest fully steerable radio telescope is called the Robert C. Byrd Green Bank Telescope, which was named after the late WV senator. Due to the observatory, the area is called the National Radio Quiet Zone. The quiet zone limits the types of radio waves. There is also no ability in the area to use cellular telephones. You have to travel around 30-60 minutes away to reach a cell signal to the town of Marlinton, Elkins or up to the Ski resort area of Snowshoe, WV. Many tourists just don't know what to do without their cell service or abundance of Wi-fi.

HIGH-FUNCTIONING AUTISM

Our wedding took place on the beautiful, hot summer day of June 23, 2012 at one of Green Bank's historical churches called Liberty Presbyterian Church, which was established in 1820. The old, white wooden church is on the same side of the road of the observatory. If we had waited one week later to get married, we would have encountered a horrific storm, the derecho of 2012, that damaged the church pretty badly. That most certainly would have caused major havoc to our day. It caused power outages for more than a week and gas shortages in the area for days.

HIGH-FUNCTIONING AUTISM

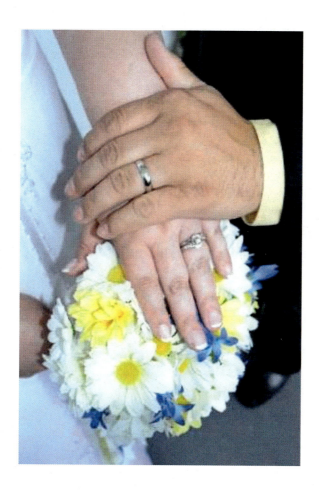

CHAPTER 5
JULY 2012 TO MAY 29, 2019

After the wedding, reception, honeymoon, and open house events were done, Karen and I continue to have many great times together, despite the challenges of life. Despite both of our chronic health issues, we could depend on each other as a newlywed couple.

Karen continued to deal with chronic back pain and other issues that were related to an early nursing career injury. I was dealing with my own health issues, including the undiagnosed autism issues.

We both got back into our lives after our honeymoon by working our jobs. I was out of work every summer due to being a public school bus driver and Karen went back to work as a home care RN right after the honeymoon.

In August 2012, I started my seventh school year driving the school bus for Guilford public school system. As time went by, the stresses as a bus driver caused more overall health issues for me. I dealt with issues that continued to get worse each year, such as students talking back at me, throwing things at me while driving the school bus, trying to get me in trouble, students fighting, walking around the bus, standing up and sitting incorrectly while the bus was in motion, and hanging out of the windows and throwing items out of the windows towards people or vehicles. I even had a child bring a dead bird on my bus. All these stresses and lack of needed support from the school system put a lot of major stress on my mind, body, and soul.

No matter what any public school supervisor would say and repeat to the bus drivers about that, "you need to keep the bus under control," it would not matter because these "children," never got any punishments for their repeated, but profoundly serious safety violations. You could write them up and somehow it would become the bus driver's fault. No matter how many times they were written up for behavioral issues, they became the same aggressors, making the bus hard to control for many of the bus drivers not only in the school system I worked in, but nationwide that has led to a national shortage of drivers due to lack of decent pay, broken up schedules and the bully and abusive behavior they deal with daily. It truly is not worth it for the amount of money you make and the lack of support you get from the supervisor.

There will be always only one adult with 30 to 72 students on the school bus. How can someone really control that many immature students when a few bad aggressors get the other children going? You cannot get them under control in an already tight route schedule and keep the pace you're supposed to follow.

It is easier to manage a few people at a time with one adult. For an example, look at school field trips with chaperones. There are more chaperones to help balance the management of a few students per chaperone, making it easier to keep things under control, unlike having a 30,000-pound vehicle full of students and a few of the same aggressors create a bigger mess on the bus, which it is a very unsafe environment for all parties inside the bus when uncalled for behavioral issues come up on a daily basis.

Therefore, the stresses of the school bus driver job and how it affected my health, created more overall health issues. It certainly didn't cause my diabetes, but it didn't help it, though. My autism also didn't help me to deal with the stresses of the unruly children and teens who misbehaved day in and day out. It was just too much. I did stay with it for the benefits and health insurance since 2008 due to becoming full-time status. It took nearly two and a half years to get full-time status and being single at the time with lack of financial resources, I did not take care of myself. It was not because I neglected to do so, it was the fact that there is a Catch 22. My bus driver's salary, which was on a full-time basis was approximately between eight to 12 dollars an hour. If you prorate my final gross wages per year, they were extremely low for the seriousness of responsibilities placed on any public school bus drivers, and, in part, contribute to their decline of overall health over a span of years.

Just an FYI, the minimum for disability to be in a person's favor from Social Security is $14,400 per year, as of 2020. That number is defined as a term that is called a lack of "gainful activity" in gross wages, but when the claim is finalized in someone's favor, it could be half of that dollar number, based on many factors on a case-by-case situation.

Some examples for any bus drivers' gross salaries in North Carolina, which are public knowledge due to being a public government employee, based on my years of working for the school system:

Example One:
$15,000 divided by 12 months equals $1,250.00 per month. Divide per month into 160 hours (40-hour week) per month equals to $7.81 per hour wages.

Example Two:
$18,000 divided by 12 months equals $1,500.00 per month. Divide per month total into 160 hours (40-hour week) per month equals to $9.38 per hour wages.

Example Three:
$20,000 divided by 12 months equals $1,666.67 per month. Divide per month total into 160 hours (40-hour week) per month equals to $10.42 per hour wages.

Example Four:
$23,000 divided by 12 months equals $1,916.67 per month. Divide per month total into 160 hours (40-hour week) per month equals to $11.98 per hour wages.

HIGH-FUNCTIONING AUTISM

Based on the above gross wages per year on average of the 12 years working for the school system, my financial health was tied to the lack of getting healthcare taken care of, as needed, which caused a perfect storm in the period that would lead to full favorable disability on January 26, 2021 by the Social Security Disability Department of the United States.

Looking back at the average gross pay per hour for the 12 years of working would be $9.98 per hour for my hourly wages. Many years in the school system had frozen pay wages and route changes per year, which affected the gross income year-by-year. Due to the many factors of low wages and the rising cost of medical care, it had put an extreme damper on my overall financial health and healthcare, along with my wife's chronic issues that required as much or more needed healthcare treatments over the years – prior to our marriage that transferred into our marriage. Only *one* health issue can cause a major *financial disaster*, which my wife and I understand, and it is part of our reality – a reality that some people may not really know how bad it was, and has been at times, and it continues to this very day.

Approaching December 2012, I started to have diabetic issues of high glucose levels, which was confirmed that I was a Type II Diabetic, and I would take only oral medications and non-insulin medications from 2012 to 2019. In addition, my health continued to get worse with my molar tooth that was a problem since the late 2000s that had a multitude of procedures like root canal, re-treatment of root canal and other treatment, which would later cause, in part, septic shock, pneumonia and staph infection in the blood in July 2018, resulting in a week-long stay at the Moses Cone Memorial Hospital, in Greensboro, North Carolina. That trauma to the body (my doctor thinks) caused me to become an insulin dependent from late 2018 to the present time.

HIGH-FUNCTIONING AUTISM

For the next few years, starting in 2013, myself and my wife would continue to do many things together, as a recent married couple to the present time.

Since I love to write sometimes, I wrote a self-publishing novel based on my feelings of September 11, 2001, which happened when I was on my church mission. I started writing my feelings after my church mission, starting in early 2003, which was finalized in early January 2014, but updated in May 2015 called *Knight Eagle: A New Breed of Superhero That Fights Terrorism*.

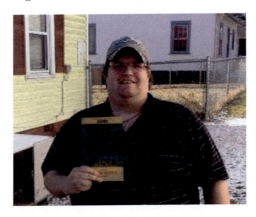

HIGH-FUNCTIONING AUTISM

Knight Eagle is a creation between a Batman and Spiderman type of superhero. He is a Green Beret and was clawed by a Bald Eagle that gives him superhuman powers by the subplot of a fictional legend called the *Legend of Knight Eagle*, which tells some Cherokee background of information. Knight Eagle lived through a domestic terrorism situation in Charlotte, under his birth name of Brandon Newman, who was a teenager at the time. There are a lot of subplots of Native Americans history. The cover below is some concept art of Knight Eagle.

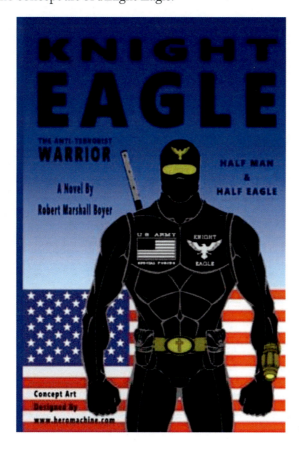

HIGH-FUNCTIONING AUTISM

A lot of influence of Knight Eagle came from my maternal grandfather Joseph Marshall Bryant as a draftee of the post-Korean War Armistice where he served with the Military Police under the direction of the United Nations Korean Communication Zone, operating under the United States Army. Other influences came from my paternal grandfather and uncle who also served in the military. Additional influences of Knight Eagle were filmmakers like James Cameron, Tim Burton and Dan Aykroyd. Mr. Aykroyd was diagnosed with high-functioning autism in the 1980s, and his obsession with law enforcement and ghost hunting helped to create the historic 1980s *Ghostbusters* franchise that continues to have growth in the upcoming, but delayed (due to the COVID-19 pandemic) feature film called *Ghostbusters: Afterlife* (2021).

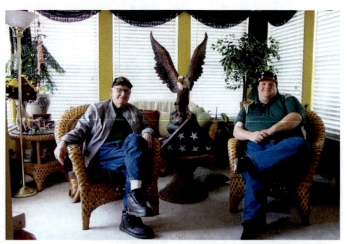

March 2014. Photo used for The Caswell Messenger in reference and influence of Marshall, as part, of the inspiration of Knight Eagle, written by his grandson Robert.

In March 2014, The Caswell Messenger, based out of Caswell County, wrote an article about Knight Eagle due to the fact that it was influenced, in part, by Caswell County native, Joseph Marshall Bryant. It was a great interview for both Mr. Boyer and Mr. Bryant.

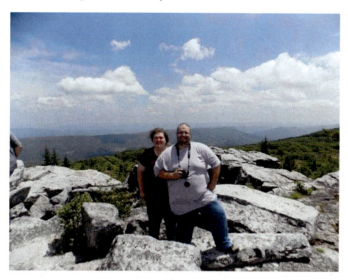

Sometime in 2015. Robert and Karen at Dolly Sods Wilderness — originally simply Dolly Sods — is a U.S. Wilderness Area in the Allegheny Mountains of eastern West Virginia, US, and is part of the Monongahela National Forest (MNF) of the U.S. Forest Service (USFS).

Since our marriage, Karen and I would frequently travel to West Virginia for quick weekend trips that were a five-to-six-hour one-way road trips to visit her family. At times we would go to historical areas like Dolly Sods and other areas of interest.

One of my narrow, obsessive-like interests is wildlife-related activities. Even though at this point in the 2015 trip to Dolly Sods and other areas, I started to not be as mobile due to my morbid obesity, uncontrolled diabetes with complications, high blood pressure and other chronic issues that were plaguing me from everyday stresses, including the undiagnosed autism, I continued to enjoy the outdoors, even if I was worn out quickly due to my fast-paced sprints, and it did not help my health issues, including some more back pain issues that were starting to become worse. Everyone has commented on why I always would walk quickly away from the group too, which is an autism trait of mine. It is natural for me to leave the group, going into my own little world. That is the nature of the beast with some autistic children and adults.

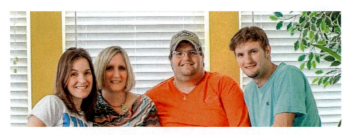

Above: Father's Day 2015. Left to Right: Seresa, Teresa, Robert, and Jared.

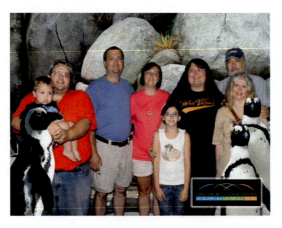

August 2015 at the Greensboro Science Center in Greensboro, NC. Left to Right is Brayden, Robert, Jason, Susan, Madeline (Maddie), Karen, Jim, and Kathy.

HIGH-FUNCTIONING AUTISM

2016 & 2017 NASCAR CUP SERIES' COCA-COLA 600
Charlotte Motor Speedway -- Memorial Day Weekend
Concord, North Carolina

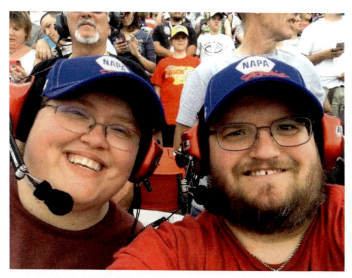

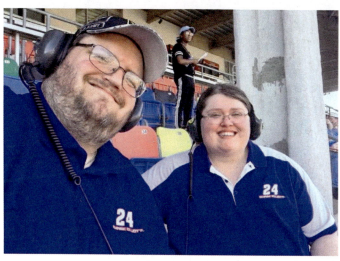

HIGH-FUNCTIONING AUTISM

2017 HOOTERS' ® CHASE ELLIOTT SHOW CAR
2017 Memorial Day Weekend
Concord, North Carolina

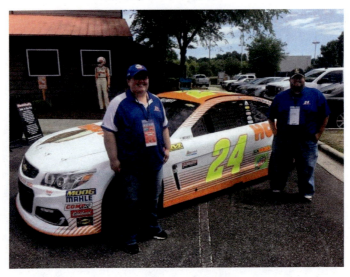

1980 STP CHEVROLET MONTE CARLO
RICHARD PETTY SHOW CAR
Martinsville Speedway (Virginia)
Spring 2018

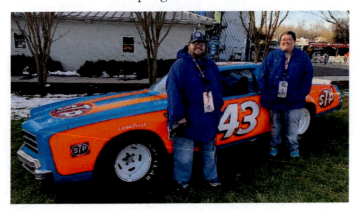

HIGH-FUNCTIONING AUTISM

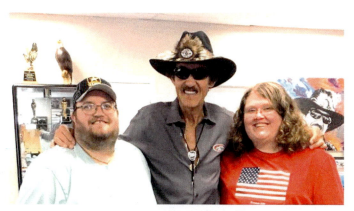

**MEETING THE KING OF NASCAR
2017 MEMORIAL DAY AT PETTY MUSEUM**

Following the annual NASCAR's historic, patriotic Coca-Cola 600 at Charlotte Motor Speedway in Concord, North Carolina, which was on the Sunday night before Memorial Day 2017, Karen and I went to the Petty Museum near our McLeansville home, which is a 30-minute drive south of McLeansville.

At the Petty Museum, Level Cross, North Carolina, Mr. Petty came in for some items to sign, which he does quite often, and the picture above was taken that day we met The King. Karen was browsing a different section of the museum and heard me say, "Hello, Richard!!" and she came over wondering what I was talking about, very surprised to see that I was talking to the "King." Richard looked at her and said, "Hi, young Lady!" to Karen, which she thought was funny. He was a genuinely nice person, like I had always thought he would be from many years of following NASCAR. My current favorite active driver is Chase Elliott #9, which is the son of NASCAR Cup Series Champion and the legendary Bill Elliott – Awesome Bill from Dawsonville. Karen always roots for Ryan Blaney #12.

HIGH-FUNCTIONING AUTISM

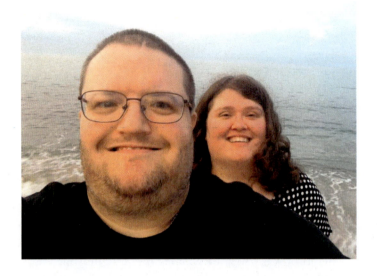

For our Fifth Wedding Anniversary – June 23, 2017 – we went to the Outer Banks of North Carolina (see picture above). we visited the Wright Brothers National Memorial at Kitty Hawk, Cape Hatteras, and other historic landmarks along the Outer Banks.

Karen, who lived most of her first 37 years of life in the West Virginia mountains, always loves to visit the beach, but not so much for me. I currently have a hard time walking on the sand from the complications of my clumsy-like motor skill deficits, and I do not handle the heat very well – it could be genetic issues that causes those problems. However, I do not mind the scenery and smells of the ocean and beach.

When I was a teenager, I went with my maternal grandfather to the Outer Banks at Ocracoke Inlet to flounder gig in the 1990s. I have great memories of gigging flounder in the sound side of the barrier island. I saw many types of marine creatures like a bathtub size sting ray and other smaller rays, including small fish when they were tailing the float with the car battery, light pole and gig pole rope. The light pole was placed just on the surface of the water to light up the sound floor, looking for those flounders to gig between their eyes. Once gigged, the gigger would slide the fish up the pole where at the other end of the pole was a rope that drug the gigged flounders in the water. Those are great memories with my grandfather in the 1990s at the Outer Banks.

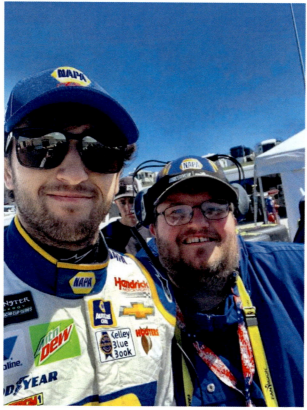

March 2018. Robert and NASCAR Cup Series driver Chase Elliott at Martinsville Speedway.

HIGH-FUNCTIONING AUTISM

From June 2017 to July 2018, my health started to decline from all aspects of life, more so with my uncontrolled glucose levels. On top of my health issues, my mental health was not the best, as I continued to struggle as a school bus driver due to the lack of support with out of control kids on the school bus that can, and do cause unsafe conditions daily – some days were worse than others.

Due to work-related stress, financial stress, and overall healthcare stress, I was thought to have a possible UTI due to burning sensations while urinating, prior to my week stay at Moses Cone Memorial Hospital (Cone). I went to the Urgent Care the day before, and the health team said it was only a UTI and treated it as such. However, when I was so lethargic and sick, my RN wife knew something was up. The next day I was in bed, sleeping all day. My sugars were in the 300's, I had a fever of 102 and just didn't look right. She called her boss and told her that she needed to get me to the ER. She took me to Cone. I had all the symptoms of Sepsis and Septic Shock such as mental status changes, low blood pressure, and rapid breathing. It was determined I was septic, had pneumonia, and a staph infection in the bloodstream. I could not breathe for a few nights, waking up gasping for air. I felt like I was going to die, and they added oxygen to my treatment regimen. I was almost admitted to the ICU, based on brief Septic Shock episodes during the week-long hospitalization. However, the medical team treatments prevented me from going to the ICU. They ended up putting me on IV antibiotics, Insulin, breathing treatments. I even went home with a PICC line, which Karen administered doses of IV antibiotics in our home at the PICC line port. In the aftermath, the post-infections caused my health to decline more. After the hospitalization I became an insulin dependent diabetic in the fall of 2018.

The health toll during the post-Septic Shock events caused more employment strain on an already stressful job

HIGH-FUNCTIONING AUTISM

as a school bus driver. I started to have some brain fog issues that effected my cognitive functions more, leading to disputes with my supervisor, which led to having a scheduled meeting with my boss's supervisor along with my union representative in January 2019. All these issues were due to the fact that my glucose levels had been through the roof since the start of the new school year. I had an eye infection and rash infection from August 2018 to December of 2018, dating back to the complications of the events that led to my hospitalization in July 2018. The nail in the coffin was the rash on one of my the legs that looked very serious, and miscommunication on what to do or not to do about calling out of work, which led to an outburst with other employees about how my supervisor did not *totally* understand my concerns. This got back to my supervisor and that led to the meeting with her supervisor, including me and my union representative.

After the January 2019 meeting, I was put on probation. But after that I ended up getting another job outside the school system as a ready-mix concrete truck driver. However, after getting hired at the new employment in February 2019, I was let go due to the difficulty of the job duties, forcing me to become unemployed by the middle of April of 2019, putting a mental and financial hardship on my household. However, I did find another job as a courier driver, but that did not last five days due to unsafe equipment and improper training that forced me to walk off in early May 2019.

Due to the hardships of failed employment from early 2019 to May 2019, I started to realize that I needed to apply for Social Security Disability. I applied and hired a disability attorney sometime around May 29, 2019, the date I officially filed the application to Social Security Disability, which would be the official date of my legal disability that was awarded on January 26, 2021.

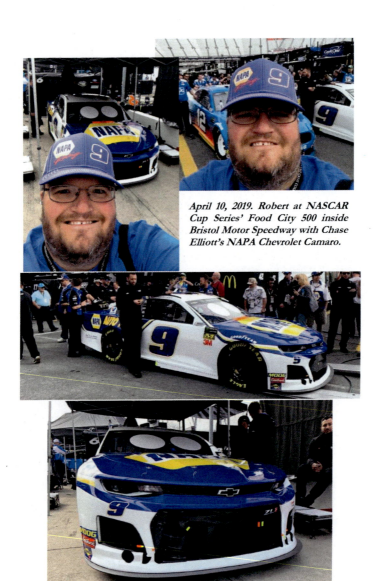

April 10, 2019. Robert at NASCAR Cup Series' Food City 500 inside Bristol Motor Speedway with Chase Elliott's NAPA Chevrolet Camaro.

HIGH-FUNCTIONING AUTISM

Top: April 28. 2019. (Back Row) Robert, Karen. Teresa. James, Seresa, Connor Robert Valdez, Jason Valdez. (Front Row) Owen Valdez.

Bottom: Labor Day Weekend 2018. Just a few months after the week-long hospitalization that was life threatening for Robert. At Darlington Raceway on Backstretch sporting a NASCAR Cups Series' Chase Elliott cap, including Karen (not pictured).

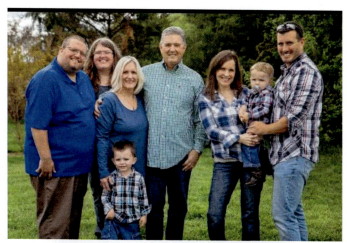

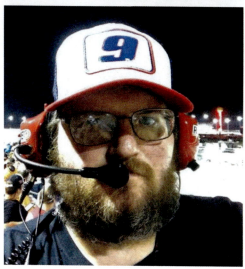

CHAPTER 6
FULLY DISABLED WITH AUTISM

After filing for disability on May 29, 2019, my focus was now getting an official diagnosis of autism. This would be a long, three-phase process. The first phase would only be with me and the psychologist. The second phase would be with the psychologist, my stepfather and mother. The last phase would be the diagnosis feedback from the completed test results that would be with the psychologist, myself, my mother and biological father.

In the meantime, in June 2019, would be the start of a cancer diagnosis for my maternal grandfather. He would be diagnosed with advanced cancer. He opted out of doing treatments because it would only spare him a few weeks of life. The cancer was so far advanced that once diagnosed, he died under hospice care inside his home on July 19, 2019. I would eulogize my grandfather at the funeral services, and I would become a part-time caregiver for my grandmother from June 2019 to July 2020. My grandmother continues to suffer from kidney failure and dementia. She needs 24/7 care, which in August 2020, she would become hospice eligible, and to this day she continues to be under hospice care in her home in Caswell County, North Carolina.

During the caregiving of Hilda Stainback Bryant, I went through the process of the disability protocols. I was seen

HIGH-FUNCTIONING AUTISM

in late 2019 by a government-provided physician for a physical examination in Greensboro, North Carolina. The physician stated to my wife and me, it does seem like I am autistic, but the physician could not address that issue due to strict protocols of the disability process. A long story short, there would be two denied statuses and my attorney would appeal the statuses, even after getting a diagnosis of autism in February 2020. However, that was a common protocol to have a denial twice, which there was a need to appeal to an Administrative Law Judge Hearing. The appeal for a court hearing was accepted in the summer of 2020, which was scheduled on December 1, 2020 with the judge.

Starting in December 2019, which would become a known fact that COVID-19 was already in the United States, based on blood test studies of COVID-19, I got sick along with my grandmother in December 2019. Once word got out about COVID-19 a few months later, there was speculation that some people were exposed to the unknown COVID-19 during the late part of 2019.

In January 2020, I was diagnosed with pre-cancerous polyps from a colonoscopy in late January 2020. In February 2020, my grandmother was hospitalized for the Flu. I was diagnosed with high-functioning autism in February 2020.

From February 2020 to July 2020, I continued to be a caregiver for my grandmother, and at the same time my wife and I would be tested a couple times for COVID-19, but the tests kept coming back as Not Detected. However, my wife kept on getting sick and has continued struggling with her asthma since her initial illness.

Finally, after issues about caregiving duties from other family members' concerns, I stopped caregiving in late July 2020, but it would end up being a blessing as I found out the following year, in late January 2021, that I had some shoulder and spinal issues from X-rays taken by the chiropractor.

HIGH-FUNCTIONING AUTISM

It was a difficult hardship from late July 2020 to early September 2020 when I was in between jobs, but with the help of Vocational Rehabilitation and Autism Society of North Carolina: Guilford County chapter, there was a job offer after months of working hard with the job coach at Autism Society, and my efforts. However, a month into the job, COVID-19 forced the company to shut down two or three times due to COVID-19 from October 2020 to December 2020, which in fact I was exposed, but the test results did not show a positive result. However, I got sick not once, but about three times. The worse episode was in early December 2020, which was after the hearing from the Administrative Law Judge on December 1, 2020.

The hearing for the disability case by the judge went well on December 1, 2020. It lasted about an hour, and the waiting game for the decision lasted until January 26, 2021 for a full favorable decision by the judge. I was considered by law – disabled – due to autism, along with the underlying issues linked to autism.

From December 4, 2020 to early February 2020, I have not been able to return to work due to some additional health issues – also it was during COVID-19. My additional health issues started with an upper respiratory illness, leading to extreme high glucose levels that sent me to the ER, twice in five days in December 2020, and finally there were more issues related to my left shoulder and spine, which was causing a lot of pain. However, the shoulder and spine were never part of the decision from the Social Security Disability's Administrative Law Judge, but for the other issues of high-functioning autism that have been addressed in the memoir.

Nevertheless, the new evidence of severe disability from the shoulder and spinal system in January 2021 affirms to me and others I am truly disabled, even prior to the recent discoveries that occurred before the fully favorable decision for myself as fully disabled by federal law.

HIGH-FUNCTIONING AUTISM

Time will tell if I can fully get back to part-time working status, but for now I have been helping with self-advocating for people with autism on my social media platforms, which you can find my Facebook page by searching for: Robert Marshall Boyer: Autism Spectrum Disorder Advocate with Autism.

My dreams are to setup a foundation in my name to help advocate for autism and/or create a scholarship for high-functioning autistic high school students.

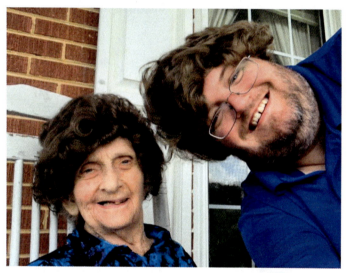

Above: August 19, 2019. Robert and (grandmother) Hilda wearing her old wigs from back in the day. Picture was taken during a caregiving day with his grandmother.

Right: A logo that was created by Robert as an advocate for any autistic individuals.

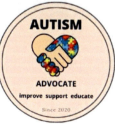

HIGH-FUNCTIONING AUTISM

AUTISM DIAGNOSIS & DNA TESTING

In February 2020, Mr. Boyer received the diagnosis that he had felt after many years of research, and his mother had come to feel that he had, which at the time was called Asperger's Disorder. However, starting in 2013 it became high-functioning autism inside the newly formed Autism Spectrum Disorder diagnosis.

In the Educational History of the official diagnosis, it stated that Mr. Boyer stayed in the home of his great-grandmother, Susie Bryant, until three years old as a daycare-like services while his parents worked. He started private speech lessons at age four and it continued to age six in kindergarten. Under Learning Disability services, starting in kindergarten, he had an Individualized Education Plan (IEP) that included occupational therapy (OT), speech therapy, accommodations for reading and math, extended testing time, and testing in a separate room, among other accommodations. He continued to have many IEP updates until his Associate's Degree in Film and Video Production Technology at Piedmont Community College-Caswell County. He was tested for auditory processing difficulties during first grade. He underwent a psychological evaluation after concerns from his teacher between first and second grade that involved issues of delayed learning differences, difficulty concentrating, articulating his thoughts, and shared suspicions that he demonstrated symptoms of AD/HD. In addition, he suffered bullying throughout his school years, causing significant distress.

In the Social Affect section of the diagnosis report, Mr. Boyer responded "incontinently in non-question bids for conversation" by "bringing up topics that are entirely unrelated to the topic" of the current conversation, and he "often interrupts to share his own thoughts, even if these are irrelevant." For eye contact issues, Mr. Boyer would look "toward" people when he talked, but eye contact was rarely involved in his conversations, often looking above the person's head. He would ask inappropriate questions (personal topics) or share personal topics to others, unaware of personal boundaries. When "he was a young child, he often pointed to express wants without coordination eye contact, but had difficulty using words to express his needs, and it was often difficult to understand his request." These "infractions" would cause frustration for Mr. Boyer "as a young child and often led to outbursts that could include destruction of nearby objects and hiding from the person he had been talking to." Mr. Boyer does not nod or shake his head during a conversation, which he never has done. His gestures are limited, and often engaged in pretend play, and he would use toys to interact with each other, such has superheroes, but he would not really talk while playing with them. By age four to five, Mr. Boyer had interest in certain objects and continues to do so, with "obsessive" frequency and intensity with a degree that is "overwhelming" that people must tell him to stop. He did not have many reciprocal friendships, "although he had only one neighborhood friend throughout elementary school." After moving to Gibsonville, he never could make any friends due to the social challenges and was often disliked and bullied. To this day, Mr. Boyer does not really have friends, but his "grandfather" was his best friend, which he recently passed away in July 2019. His grandfather was patient with him, trying to build and "teach appropriate social skills" for his grandson.

Some of the restricted or repetitive behaviors that Mr. Boyer struggles with are shakes, twists, and flapping his hands with excitement, including "full body mannerisms that consists of shuffling his feet and repeatedly standing up and sitting down when others are talking about a topic that does not interest him, or when he is required to sit" for any extensive amount of time, such as when he was attending his grandfather's funeral, he could not stand in line and would walk around the room interacting with others. When there is a topic he is interested in, he is "like a different person" due to the topic that suits him (narrow, obsessive-like topics).

Mr. Boyer, Ms. Gentry and Ms. Boyer showed that Mr. Boyer had consistently endorsed "ongoing symptoms of both social impairment and restricted and repetitive behaviors that interfered with (Mr. Boyer's) overall functioning…including difficulty engaging in reciprocal social relationships and difficulty understanding social boundaries, as well as ongoing circumscribed interests (news, weather, firetrucks, airplanes, mold, running water) and hand mannerisms (flapping hands, etc.). Reports across raters are consistent with behaviors observations from this evaluation indicating that (Mr. Boyer) experiences ongoing symptoms of social impairments and restricted and repetitive behaviors that interfere with his overall functions. Notably, (Mr. Boyer) has had a diagnosis of AD/HD since his early childhood, as well as diagnoses of persistent depressive disorder, central processing auditory disorder, and specific learning disability. These diagnoses do not adequately explain the extent of (Mr. Boyer's) difficulty engaging in reciprocal social interactions, nor his restricted and repetitive behaviors. Additionally, it is believed that (Mr. Boyer's) persistent symptoms of depression is likely related to the extent of his difficulty engaging in reciprocal social interactions. Taken

HIGH-FUNCTIONING AUTISM

together, (Mr. Boyer) meets criteria of Autism Spectrum Disorder."

HIGH-FUNCTIONING AUTISM

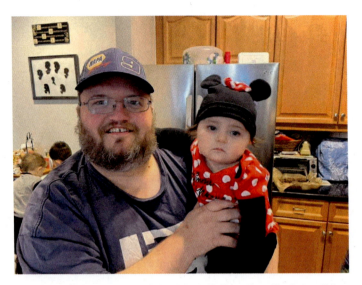

February 2021. Robert with Hope Marie Valdez, niece. Background is Connor and Owen Valdez, nephews.

On March 1, 2021, I got a call from Brenner Children's Hospital at Wake Forest Baptist Hospital in Winston-Salem concerning the DNA results indicated that may be connected to autism and other developmental disorders. The results at this time there was no DNA connection to autism. However, since new genes are always being discovered that are linked to autism, that I will need to call the hospital back in two years for a follow-up for any updates on the genetic research. Despite the news from Brenner, there is hope that one day there will be more genetic breakthroughs that may be connected to my DNA. Until then, I'm grateful for the crazy roller-coaster ride in my first 40 years of my life that has led me to this point.

Life deals you a certain hand of playing cards. You just have to believe and continue to have hope that life will get better as things continue to progress.

HIGH-FUNCTIONING AUTISM

NATIONAL AUTISM ASSOCIATION
Fact Sheet on Autism
https://nationalautismassociation.org/resources/autism-fact-sheet/

What is Autism?

- Autism is a bio-neurological developmental disability that generally appears before the age of 3.
- Autism impacts the normal development of the brain in the areas of social interaction, communication skills, and cognitive function. Individuals with autism typically have difficulties in verbal and non-verbal communication, social interactions, and leisure or play activities.
- Individuals with autism often suffer from numerous co-morbid medical conditions which may include: allergies, asthma, epilepsy, digestive disorders, persistent viral infections, feeding disorders, sensory integration dysfunction, sleeping disorders, and more.
- Autism is diagnosed four times more often in boys than girls. Its prevalence is not affected by race, region, or socio-economic status. Since autism was first diagnosed in the U.S. the incidence has climbed to an alarming one in 54 children in the U.S.
- Autism itself does not affect life expectancy, however research has shown that the mortality risk among individuals with autism is twice as high as the general population, in large part due to drowning and other accidents.
- Currently there is no cure for autism, though with <u>early intervention and treatment</u>, the diverse symptoms related to autism can be greatly improved and in some cases completely overcome.

HIGH-FUNCTIONING AUTISM

Autism Facts & Stats
- Autism now affects 1 in 54 children; over half are classified as having an intellectual disability or borderline intellectual disability.
- Boys are four times more likely to have autism than girls.
- About 40% of children with autism do not speak. About 25%–30% of children with autism have some words at 12 to 18 months of age and then lose them. Others might speak, but not until later in childhood
- Autism greatly varies from person to person (no two people with autism are alike).
- The rate of autism has steadily grown over the last twenty years.
- Comorbid conditions often associated with autism include Fragile X, allergies, asthma, epilepsy, bowel disease, gastrointestinal/digestive disorders, persistent viral infections, PANDAS, feeding disorders, anxiety disorder, bipolar disorder, ADHD, Tourette Syndrome, OCD, sensory integration dysfunction, sleeping disorders, immune disorders, autoimmune disorders, and neuroinflammation.
- Autism is the fastest growing developmental disorder, yet most underfunded.
- A 2008 Danish Study found that the mortality risk among those with autism was nearly twice that of the general population.
- Children with autism do progress – early intervention is key.
- Autism is treatable, not a hopeless condition.

HIGH-FUNCTIONING AUTISM

QUESTIONS AND ANSWERS SECTION WITH ROBERT MARSHALL BOYER

Question 1
Did you speculate that you had an undiagnosed autism situation and understood what autism is?

Yes, I did.

Speculation of Undiagnosed Autism: *When I reviewed my healthcare records, along with memory and current behaviors, the "red flags" were always there. Times have changed a lot since the 1980s when I was diagnosed with other learning disorders including speech and language delay (circa 1983), meltdowns (everyone speculated it was more like temper tantrums), over reaction to stimuli/sensitivity issues, texture issues like the dislike of fruits, central auditory processing disorder, attention deficit/hyperactivity disorder, fine motor skills deficits and gross motor skills deficits. I was never diagnosed for what would have been Asperger's Disorder (now known as high-functioning autism).*

Understanding of autism: *I knew what autism was at the time, as I was trying to figure out on why I had certain behaviors that were linked to me being socially awkward.*

Question 2
Are there things that really bother you or frustrate/annoy you?

Yes. Stimuli of certain sounds smells, and other sensations do bother me, but not every day is the same. It depends on each situation. My body gets overwhelmed at night, most of the time, which seems to be over-stimuli of my functions. I start to stem (repetitive movements) like pacing, rubbing my feet together, hands together, almost like hyperactivity, but it is due to over stimuli when things start to bother me, frustrate me, and annoy

HIGH-FUNCTIONING AUTISM

me. However, these issues do not always happen at night, it can be anytime without any warning at all. Certain texture and taste of food bothers me – I do not like fruit in general.

Question 3
Are there things that you are afraid of?

Yes. Mostly how to make ends meet due to the lack of resources that cost so much money, and I am now officially disabled by federal law as of January 26, 2021 due to autism, among the other underlying issues with it. Fear is the main underlying issue that triggers a lot of anxiety, depression, and stress, which all are intertwined with autism. It is a complicated situation, which causes intense fear from me quite often.

Question 4
What kinds of things are you really good at? Can you play music or sing, for example?

I am good at filming and video editing. I once sung in middle school until my voice changed, and I can make up melodies with guitar and piano, but have a hard time remembering what I created. I took lessons on guitar for a few years, but due to frustrations I gave it up. I am good at building things like electronics. I can remember details of statistics like sports, events, and dates. I am good on the computer and good with children, adults, and elderly who may have cognitive issues.

Question 5
What are your hobbies/ favorite things to do?

I love the outdoors (hunting and fishing mostly) but love to be around mother nature. I love watching movies* and going to NASCAR races with my wife. Other interests are related to film and videoing, photoshop and working on any technological subjects like computers and gadgets. I love video games, especially NASCAR racing games.

HIGH-FUNCTIONING AUTISM

*My favorite genres of movies are action, war-themed and based on true events.

Question 6
Do you have a job? What do you do?

Yes. Currently, before I got sick in early December 2020, I worked at a pre-assemble warehouse that involves adults with autism or other developmental cognitive issues. My job title is production worker and driver. My main duties are assembling equipment, prepare them on skids for shipment and drive the box truck, when needed. Depending on the outcome of my current health issues, I am not sure what will happen. What will happen in returning to work again? Time will tell.

Question 7
Where do you live?

I live in the rural town of McLeansville. It is a few miles east of Greensboro, North Carolina. I live in the northern part of the town with my wife and two cats.

Question 8
Do you remember what it was like when you were a kid? Remember what it was like to be a kid?

Yes, I remember what it was like when I was a kid. I do not remember the struggles as much but do remember the events of some evaluations that involved psychological and medical issues. I had a childhood friend that lived down the road from me before I moved away from Burlington. After that, I was a loner, outcast due to my social awkwardness that played a part in my struggles with my learning disabilities. Middle and high school were the worst part of being a kid due to many of my issues. That is when I gained weight, but I was a picky eater – never liked fruit. I was not as active as a kid, and still am not. There are many more things that I do remember, but it is all connected to the struggles I had, but I did have many fond memories too as a kid – it was not all that bad as a kid. But could have been better in areas of my childhood.

HIGH-FUNCTIONING AUTISM

A few good memories as a kid, including playing sports as a pre-high school kid like baseball and soccer. I was a manager for JV men's basketball, Varsity men's basketball and football, including one year playing football in 11th grade at Eastern Guilford High School. The coaches were my friends, not many of my peers.

Question 9
How many friends do you have currently?

Less than a dozen "friends," but have "buddies" that I hang out with. My friends are my family members. Due to my social awkwardness, it has always been a struggle to keep "friends" unless they knew that I had some issues, and they overlooked my awkwardness.

Question 10
Do you have any brothers or sisters? Where do they live?

Yes. I have a little biological sister that is 30 months younger than me. I have a half-brother that is 10 years younger than me from my stepfather and mother's relationship. I have two stepsisters from my stepfather's previous marriage. Then I have one stepsister from my stepmother's previous marriage. They all live in North Carolina, within 30 minutes to an hour away from my home.

Question 11
Do you get along with other people? No fighting?

That depends. If people do not understand my struggles of autism, it does cause frustrations in overall relationships like friends, family, social, employment and business. Frustrations would build up and there were verbal arguments, sometimes objects would get damaged from a frustration breakdown and/or meltdown, such as throwing, punching, and tearing up objects. Very rarely would there be a physical-like fight that may break out.

Question 12

HIGH-FUNCTIONING AUTISM

Do you find it difficult to spend time with other people?

Yes, all the time. It all goes back to the issues of autism. Family and close family friends, for the most part, understand or adapt to my issues, but they can have times of frustration due to my struggles, causing lack of spending time with others. It is hard on everyone at times, which that is why I only spend time with those who understand me more than the "social circles" that cause anxiety for me.

Question 13
Do you know of anyone else in your family who has autism too?

Yes, I do.

Question 14
What was it like going to school? Did you get to sit in a classroom with other kids or did you have to go to a room with differently abled kids?

It was not a good situation. I was bullied a lot due to my struggles. I was an easy target. I was jumped in the high school restroom and had a seat pulled away from me during high school graduation by a classmate.

I was in special education classes and normal classes throughout my years in school. The non-special education classes were much harder to deal with due to my slow nature of me trying to learn and keeping up with the pace of sessions daily in school. I fell behind a lot. I had an IEP (Individualized Education Program).

Question 15
What kinds of things do you think are funny? Who makes you laugh?

HIGH-FUNCTIONING AUTISM

Funny movies make me laugh. However, I do not get jokes that much due to autism. A lot of famous comedians make me laugh, as well as some family members and friends.

Question 16
What is relaxing to you?

Movies, editing videos, creating photoshop projects, outdoor activities such as hiking, the mountains, the beach, going to sports events, especially NASCAR races. And of course, spending time with my family members.

Question 17
What do you dream about most?

Being more successful in life. Advocate for autism. Hoping to start a foundation and/or scholarship fund in my name to help those that need help. I want to use my experience to help others improve better than I did in life by trying to help others not go through what I did due to not getting diagnosed until I was nearly 40-years-old.

Question 18
What do you do when people make fun of you or do not have nice things to say about people with autism?

I laugh or joke it off about me personally, at first, but when anyone says negative things about autistic people, I tell them straight up how it makes me feel, and I will educate them about what I have been through, and what other autistic people are dealing with.

Question 19
What is the meanest thing anybody ever said or did to you?

HIGH-FUNCTIONING AUTISM

There are many things that I can think of like the events in high school, but when I was a school bus driver for 12 years I think back to when the students on the bus preyed on my issues and they would bully me, cuss at me, throw things at me, try to get me in trouble with school officials, and other issues that caused much stress.

Question 20
Is there anything else you want to share about your autism diagnosis?

Yes, I do. This journey took nearly four decades. It was a rough, long road for me, my family, and the healthcare teams over the years. I do not fault anything during the diagnosis process, but there are "What Ifs" all the time due to the missed years of getting the proper treatments that would have helped me succeed better in my first 39 years, of my life. I feel like I had missed opportunities due to being underdiagnosed, misdiagnosed or undiagnosed. This memoir was not only therapy for me, but a way to share and advocate for those who are struggling like me, hoping they will find the needed help if they have never been diagnosed within the autism spectrum. If you, or a loved one, feels like you have any "red flags" of development, there are more resources out there than there were in the 1980s to 2010s that can help with early interventions, or in some cases get you on the right track if you are an adult with an undiagnosed form of autism. In conclusion, I know what it feels like not being diagnosed with autism and the struggles of not getting proper treatment, and the missed opportunities that happened over the years that could have made life more successful. It is through my sincere hope, dream, and desire that the medical and psychological fields will work together to help diagnose any form of autism for today and tomorrow a lot faster than it took with my case that took four decades to get the proper diagnosis of autism spectrum disorder – high-functioning autism.

HIGH-FUNCTIONING AUTISM

HIGH-FUNCTIONING AUTISM

ABOUT THE AUTHOR:
ROBERT MARSHALL BOYER

Robert Marshall Boyer (Germany spelling of *Beyer*), with an overall ancestry roots from United Kingdom, Sweden and German, was born on October 16, 1980 to the parents of Michael Robert Boyer and Teresa Lynn Bryant in the City of Burlington, North Carolina. His father's background ancestry is Pennsylvania Dutch (Germany) on his parents' side, and his mother background ancestry is from Sweden and Wales (UK). He attended Hilcrest Elementary, briefly Gibsonville Elementary, McLeansville Middle and Eastern Guilford High School. In high school he was a basketball and football manager, including one year a football player. He was an outstanding senior in his yearbook. He served a two-year, volunteer mission in Iowa, Missouri, and Illinois for The Church of Jesus Christ of Latter-day Saints. He graduated with a GPA of 3.5 in the Film and Video Production Technology's Associate's Program at Piedmont Community College-Caswell Campus with an Outstanding Student award in the program. He worked for the public school system for 12 years as a school bus driver and a caregiver for his grandmother for a year. He has been married since June 23, 2012 to his wife Karen and has two cats. They are currently living in McLeansville, North Carolina.

HIGH-FUNCTIONING AUTISM

HIGH-FUNCTIONING AUTISM

ABOUT THE AUTHOR:
TERESA BRYANT GENTRY

Teresa Bryant Gentry was born as Teresa Lynn Bryant to Hilda Marie Stainback and Joseph Marshall Bryant on November 4, 1958. She attended schools in Burlington, North Carolina, including Cummings High School, with the honor of Salutatorian in her Class of 1977. She attended Elon College (Elon University) for two years before transferring to Brigham Young University (BYU), which is a church-owned university of The Church of Jesus Christ of Latter-day Saints, and she is a member of that church. While attending BYU, she met her ex-husband Michael "Mike" Robert Boyer, and they have two children, Robert Marshall Boyer, and Seresa Marie Boyer. After they divorced, they remarried other spouses. Ms. Gentry and her current husband had Jared Watkins Gentry. She retired as a government contractor for a Fortune 500 company. She enjoys thrift shopping with Debbie Poteat and others. She took her mother out thrift shopping for many years that were simply called "girlfriend day" every Wednesday. Due to her mother's declining health, the mother-daughter tradition, which included Ms. Bryant eating a "heavy with chili and light of the slaw" hotdog from Zack's Hotdogs had to stop. Ms. Gentry spends time with her family and grandchildren. Ms. and Mr. Gentry have been doing a service mission for their local church's Bishop's Storehouse (food bank) and food storage center for the last few years.

HIGH-FUNCTIONING AUTISM

HIGH-FUNCTIONING AUTISM

ABOUT THE EDITOR:
KAREN RAY BOYER, RN

Karen Melissa Ray was born in Ronceverte, West Virginia on August 22, 1980 to James and Kathy Ray. She has an older brother, Jason, who is married to Susan. They have two children. Karen wasn't able to have her own children and loves them to pieces. Karen attended schools in the towns of Green Bank and Dunmore, WV. Graduating from Pocahontas County High School in 1998. She attended Marshall University in Huntington, WV for one year before eventually attending Davis & Elkins College. She started Nursing school in 2000 and graduated with an Associates of Science in Nursing in May of 2002. She was the treasurer of DESNA (D&E student nurses association). She has worked in many settings as a Registered nurse such as the hospital, juvenile center, skilled nursing facility, hospice, home health care and as an inbound call center nurse. In her spare time, she makes art and resin crafts, reads a lot of books and likes to go on random road trips and visit the beach with her husband. She resides in McLeansville, NC with her husband Robert and two cats.

HIGH-FUNCTIONING AUTISM

Made in the USA
Columbia, SC
24 August 2021